"A truly remarkable book with riveting and powerful stories. Real healing involves more than pills and surgery. Dr. Chris Gilbert with her compassion and masterful insights uncovers the root cause of seemingly inexplicable and mystifying symptoms of many illnesses. She teaches us how to have our patients discover the hidden cause of what ails them, address it and realize spectacular and long-lasting benefits. This book is a must-read."

**SANJIV CHOPRA, MD, MACP**
Professor of Medicine Harvard Medical School
Best-selling author of many books, including
*The Big Five: Five Simple Things You Can Do to Live a Longer,
Healthier Life* and *Live Better, Live Longer*
Motivational Speaker

"Useful advice from an unconventional physician and a knowledgeable neuroscientist, a brilliant pair who provide insight into emotions and effects of stress that trigger physical illness. The uniqueness of this book is that Dr. Gilbert provides the medical diagnosis, and Dr. Haseltine provides explanation based on fundamental neuroscience. A splendid combination!"

**DR. RITA COLWELL**
Former President of the American Association for the Advancement
of Science. Distinguished University Professor at
The University of Maryland and Johns Hopkins
Bloomberg School of Public Health

"Dr. Chris Gilbert and neuroscientist Eric Haseltine have produced a book full of canny insights into the importance of stress as a cause of disease, which is both useful and intriguing."

**NORMAN E. ROSENTHAL, MD**
Clinical Professor of Psychiatry at
Georgetown University School of Medicine
Author of *Super Mind* (Tarcher Perigree 2016)

"If you want to understand what Mind/Body medicine really is, then read *The Listening Cure*. This is a curiously terrific book. It draws you in and doesn't let you go."

# THE
# LISTENING CURE

# THE
# LISTENING
# CURE

HEALING SECRETS OF AN UNCONVENTIONAL DOCTOR

by Chris Gilbert, MD, PhD
with Eric Haseltine, PhD

SELECTBOOKS
NEW YORK

This edition published by SelectBooks, Inc.
For information address SelectBooks, Inc., New York, New York.
First Edition
ISBN 978-1-59079-437-1

Library of Congress Cataloging-in-Publication Data

Names: Gilbert, Chris, [date]- author. | Haseltine, Eric, author.
Title: The listening cure : healing secrets of an unconventional doctor / by Chris Gilbert, MD, PhD, with Eric Haseltine, PhD.
Description: First edition. | New York : SelectBooks, Inc., [2017]
Identifiers: LCCN 2017012069 | ISBN 9781590794371 (pbk. book : alk. paper)
Subjects: LCSH: Mind and body therapies. | Mind and body.
Classification: LCC RC489.M53 G55 2017 | DDC 616.89/14–dc23 LC record available at https://lccn.loc.gov/2017012069

Interior Design by Pauline Neuwirth, Neuwirth & Associates, Inc.

Manufactured in the United States of America

10 9 8 7 6 5 4 3 2 1

"Listen to your body! It talks to you through cravings, pleasures, orgasms, aches and pains, and many more ways. Give it a voice, and you'll understand its needs, likes, and dislikes. This is key to a healthy, balanced, and happy life."

—Chris Elisabeth Gilbert, MD, PhD

# Contents

# Preface

How is suppressed anger related to back pain?
Why do feelings of helplessness promote obesity?
What is the connection between guilt and chronic fatigue?
How can an unhappy marriage cause psoriasis?

I have been a physician for over thirty years and have practiced medicine all over the world: from a state-of the-art UCLA hospital in Los Angeles to primitive conditions in a hospital tent in a Mauritanian refugee camp at the Mali border during my time with Doctors Without Borders. My experiences have led me to view disease and the curing of disease in a very different, unconventional way from many doctors.

I have learned that many of the most common ailments that send patients to doctors, such as joint pain, abdominal pain, fatigue, sexual disorders, obesity, skin rashes, and headaches are not purely physical problems. Instead, they have their origin in intense and extreme, but also suppressed emotions from internal conflicts deep within the human psyche.

In my view, burying strong feelings like anger, frustration, fear, sadness, loss, lust, and envy can cause illness.

For this reason I have found that the route to healing many ordinary maladies begins not with the physical side of their ailments but with my patients' minds. In many cases, the physical symptoms are mere surface manifestations—the tip of the ice-berg—that signal that something is very wrong and must be at-tended to. But the healing in these instances can never be permanent until the patient's feelings of stress and strain from internal struggles are dealt with.

Unfortunately, the overwhelming majority of family practice and internal medicine physicians do not spend much time deal-ing with their patients' inner lives. They focus on the external, physical symptoms and not much else. The result is that patients are treated with prescription drugs, most of them painkillers. They undergo expensive tests and sometimes surgery that treat the symptoms they suffer from, but do nothing to heal the under-lying causes of the illness. All too often, cures achieved in this manner are temporary or force the patient to suffer debilitating side effects of drugs. These methodologies, the fruit of modern medical practice, may help alleviate discomfort and pain, but, tragically, often ignore and rarely fix the root causes of these ill-nesses. The underlying emotional health problem is almost never diagnosed, let alone treated.

Here's a remarkable statistic: It's been estimated that eighty percent of illnesses treated by primary care physicians are related to stress, behavioral, or emotional problems—exactly the kinds of problems that are almost never addressed!

In looking for ways to locate these underlying sources of illness, I have learned that neither Western medicine nor Eastern medi-cine have all the answers. But after many years of exploring outside the conventions of modern medicine, I have found better, uncon-ventional ways to observe, diagnose, and treat my patients.

I have developed a new kind of practice that looks behind the symptoms for the true origins and causes of illness and treats those causes effectively and efficiently, usually without drugs and their side effects. I have, as a consequence, been able to produce unexpected cures in my patients.

When I examine a patient I first look at the purely physical aspects of the ailment. If the problem is apparent—maybe it's an injury, a crushed vertebra or maybe a bacterial infection—then I know what kinds of drugs or other conventional therapies to order. However, when my examination reveals no apparent reason for the problem, or when the apparent reason seems too minor to cause a high level of chronic pain, I turn to my unconventional methods—my healing secrets.

I have come to believe that the information I need to cure my patients is already inside them, and I need to discover it. My source of information is the body itself, in the signals it gives us through the symptoms of our illnesses. I have found that, with some coaxing, we can get our body to give up its secrets and point us to the true source of illness. From there, true, lasting cures are possible.

I have, in effect, learned to decipher the language of the body to understand what it is trying to tell us when illnesses arise. I do this by giving the body a "voice" through engaging my patient in guided dialogues, dramatizations, arguments, role playing, visualizations, and art creation. Through these techniques, undiscovered emotions such as anger, rage, frustration and fear and debilitating conflicts are revealed that are directly related to my patients' ailments. Once these are recognized, they can be treated and possibly eliminated—along with the physical ailments that have become their outward manifestation.

You have a right to ask how I can possibly believe that the body has its own language and that there is a way to communicate with it. Or that the body really "speaks." The answer is that our physical bodies and our nervous systems and our brains are all one beautifully complex, connected organism. Everything that happens to us both in our interactions with the world as well as deep within our bodies is noticed and remembered by our brains. By coaxing our "bodies" to speak, I am actually tapping into stored memories and unconscious feelings that are intimately connected body to mind, mind to body.

By using my healing secrets such as playacting and visualizations, I am able to draw out the body's complaints to reveal the deep, underlying cause of illness, and bring long-lasting health and happiness to my patient.

There is a scientific basis for understanding the efficacy of these healing methods.

My coauthor, Dr. Eric Haseltine, a prominent neuroscientist, has helped me in the course of this book to present the hard-science biological and psychological factors that explain the success of my healing secrets.

Why am I writing this book? And why should you read it?

Having used these unconventional practices over the years with countless patients in my private medical practice, I now want to share my secrets with you. My mission is to explain my methods to the best of my ability so that many people all over the world can benefit from them.

I will take you on a fascinating journey into the lives of my patients, revealing how I treat and cure them. And I will show you how you can apply my methods for yourself and for your loved ones. My healing techniques will help you to head off illness, and they will help you understand the nature and the source of your illness and what to do about it.

Of course, the information in this book cannot cover all maladies and every patient. But if you have been dissatisfied with the way doctors have treated you; if you are suffering from chronic, unexplained pain in your joints, including pain in your back, or in your abdomen; if you have chronic fatigue syndrome, depression, anxiety, obesity, headaches, skin rashes, or sexual problems; if all the tests your doctor gave you reveal nothing or only very minor abnormalities, this book is for you. It might transform your life. If you have recurrent infections, or even cancer, you will learn to listen to your body and begin to understand its reactions to chemotherapy, radiation therapy, or other conventional forms of treatment that may be necessary for your recovery.

The healing secrets I reveal in this book will allow you, perhaps for the first time, to be in touch with your body. You will learn to listen to your body, understand what it is saying, and uncover the deep sources of your ailments. My healing techniques will open the way to long-lasting cures that may have eluded you in the past, cures that are beyond the scope of conventional Western medicine.

We hope you will use these secrets well. And we wish you good health.

# NOTE TO READERS

*The Listening Cure* is based on the professional experiences of Dr. Chris Gilbert in treating patients in her own medical practice, and the experiences of Dr. Eric Haseltine in treating patients in his own therapy practice. The book is told from Dr. Gilbert's point of view. However, no real patients (or their friends and families) are named or depicted in the book. All such names and other identifying details are fictitious, and all patients and case histories depicted in the book are composites based on the experiences of multiple individuals. The conversations between the authors and the composite patients are inspired by real conversations but have been composed for use in this book. For these reasons, any similarity between the patients and case histories in this book and any real individuals is strictly coincidental.

Throughout this book, you will find examples of patient experiences that are typical to those of real patients whom Dr. Gilbert and Dr. Haseltine have treated. The authors are sharing these examples to expand the thinking and enhance the knowledge of the reader with the goal of improving physical health and psychological well-being. But it is important for you to keep in mind that no book can take the place of a consultation between a patient and his or her physician, therapist, or other appropriate healthcare professional, and this book is not intended to do so. Each person will have his or her own unique physical and mental health issues, and some of the information and advice in this book may not be appropriate for a particular reader.

The authors have made every effort to present information that they believed to be accurate and complete at the time of publication. However, you should satisfy yourself that the information is up-to-date by consulting the professionals who are responsible for your health care.

For all of the reasons discussed above, this book is not intended to assist the reader in diagnosing or treating any medical or psychological condition, and does not create a physician-patient or therapist-patient relationship between you and either of the authors. You should consult your physician, therapist, or other appropriate health-care professional before relying on or using any of the content of this book (or any other book).

CHRIS GILBERT, MD, PHD, and ERIC HASELTINE, PHD

# 1

# Scream, Cry, and Laugh Your Way to Good Health

"**I** HATE YOU! I hate you!! I hate you!!!

Cynthia's voice became louder and louder as she hit with more and more force.

"You're a workaholic!!! You don't care about me anymore!!! You just want sex from me—no matter what hour of the night you come home. You've destroyed all the good we had in our marriage—all the love and romance and caring. I am not even attracted to you anymore!!! F... you! F... you!! F... you!!! Cynthia starts hitting again.

Cynthia's beautiful green eyes are full of tears. Her lovely face is bright red, flushed with anger. A slender women, her long auburn hair swings left and right, as her arms pump and her clenched fists smash into the plump pillows I've placed on my examination table.

Her fists are moving faster and faster, and she looks a sight—a lovely, well-dressed woman in an elegant blue dress punching those poor defenseless pillows.

But this is the moment I've been waiting for. Cynthia is letting her guard down and is allowing whatever she is feeling, and may not be aware of, to come up to the surface. She has managed to trust the process I've offered her that allows her to be vulnerable and nonjudgmental and to commit to saying what is true in the moment without any self-censuring. I am so proud of her.

Suddenly she laughs. It's a loud laugh, coming from deep inside. It sounds like a nervous reaction after an intense release of energy.

I ask, "What is going on? How are you feeling now? How intense is the pain in your throat?"

Tears come to her eyes. After taking a deep breath, she declares, "Dr. Chris, this feels really good! The pain in my throat doesn't feel so bad anymore!!!"

I am thrilled, so glad that she is feeling better.

My work with Cynthia is an example of the unconventional way I interact with my patients in order to accurately diagnose and treat their ailments. When faced with symptoms such as Cynthia's, that could be due to stress, I have found ways to release the destructive, bottled-up emotions that people keep inside themselves—emotions that may be the source of their illness. In the case of anger, one way is to make people actively bang on pillows to direct the destructive energy towards the pillows rather than keeping it buried inside and having it turn against them.

"Bottled-up emotion" is not just a convenient phrase; there is a great deal of truth in the words. When we suppress negative feelings, such as anger, fear, and hurt as Cynthia has done, our brain's limbic system goes into action. It sends out signals that make the adrenal glands release stress hormones such as adrenaline and cortisol that are supposed to prepare our bodies physically to deal with difficult or dangerous situations. This is a great process if, say, we are being attacked and have to defend ourselves or run away. But in everyday life, it can cause more problems than it solves.

What happens is that cortisol depresses our immune system, making us open to infection. Our muscles, bathed in excess cortisol and adrenaline, get more excitable and irritable, leading to muscle tension and spasms in various parts of the body. All this is occurring inside us even as our conscious minds have moved on, and we may no longer feel actively angry or upset or fearful.

This is what is happening to Cynthia, and as we'll see in the course of the book, to many of the other patients I have been able to cure with my unconventional methods.

If we are ill, recent research suggests that emotional problems related to behavioral problems such as bottled-up anger are, as in Cynthia's case, the root cause of our being sick. It's been estimated that around eighty percent of visits to primary care physicians are due to symptoms ultimately caused by stress or emotional problems. So, while we may not have Cynthia's chronically sore throat, but are not feeling well for another reason, the odds are overwhelming that Cynthia's case is highly relevant to what we are experiencing.

Now let's see how I identified Cynthia's problem and dealt with it.

Cynthia has come to see me for chronic throat pain that started two years prior to her first visit. It began after an argument with her husband over his refusal to take time to play with their kids on weekends. He is a hardworking man dedicated to his job and with little time to devote to his family.

Cynthia began to feel that her throat was swollen, that perhaps there was a growth in it causing her pain and discomfort. Over time her symptoms got worse, sometimes even preventing her from swallowing.

She saw many physicians: An ear, nose, and throat physician performed a larynx endoscopy, looking for a lump next to her vocal chords. Another one ordered a neck CT scan, looking for a mass that might be outside her throat, pressing on it. A gastroenterologist did an upper endoscopy looking at her esophagus and stomach with a camera to rule out cancer or an ulcer. The test revealed nothing abnormal. Nobody found anything wrong with her. Her primary care physician gave her hope that a steroid spray would bring her relief, but it didn't work. She tried numerous medications and supplements, but none were able to alleviate her pain, which had slowly been increasing for about two months.

Then one day she comes to see me.

As she enters my examination room, I immediately notice that she looks very distressed. As we greet each other, I hear a voice that is soft, but more importantly, it sounds very weak.

After examining her, I say, "Cynthia, I'd like to try something you might find unusual at first. I'd like you to give your throat a voice. If your throat could talk without being censored or judged, what would it say? Remember, this would not be *you* talking, it would be your *throat*."

She looks at me quizzically, but I can also see that she is desperate enough to try anything.

Now, a little sound begins to emanate from her throat: "Dr. Chris, I don't know! I am so weak and tired! It feels like I have a lump in me! It's painful!"

Now I want to get her to bypass the controlling consciousness and get in touch with her body's sensations that are closer to her unconscious. "Okay," I say. "Throat! Tell me more!"

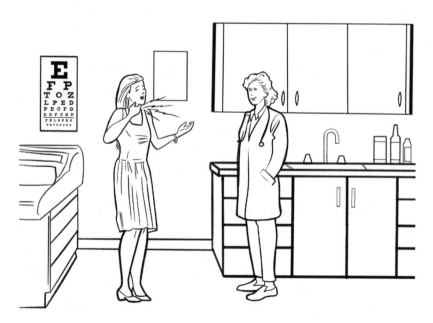

*Cynthia comes to the office complaining of chronic throat pain.*
*Dr. Chris: "Is there anything your throat wants to say?"*

Cynthia is responsive, "It feels big to me, like a ping-pong ball. It is round."

I ask her, "Anything else? Say whatever comes to mind! It doesn't even need to make sense to you! Ready, set, go! Talk!"

In order to keep open that bridge from the body to the unconscious, I need Cynthia to talk immediately without thinking since thinking would bring her consciousness into the equation.

"I have a big ball of knots inside of me! Tense knots! I want to get rid of them! I am so angry I could scream!" Jumping back to her conscious mind, Cynthia suddenly apologizes for her outburst, "Oh! I'm sorry! I didn't want to say that! That was horrible!"

Before the apology, Cynthia has yelled out a key sentence: "I am so angry I could scream!" Her conscious mind doesn't want to admit that, but her body does. Her outburst sounds like a deep truth from her unconscious but is immediately judged by her conscious mind to be "horrible." Over the years, I have learned to pay attention and respect what the unconscious says through the body. Now I have to confirm what she just said.

"Cynthia, that was not horrible! That sounded real! Check within yourself . . . Was there some truth to it?"

"Yes," she replies in the small, shy voice again.

"Okay, Cynthia, what I am hearing is that your body is so angry, it could scream. Is that right?"

"Yes," says the small, shy voice again.

The shy voice indicates to me that the unconscious body is present but is very weak, completely dominated by the controlling conscious mind. Yet, the deep reason for her throat pain has to be found in the unconscious mind, which is very tentatively speaking out for itself.

"Cynthia, I want to hear more about what your body wants to say to us. What else would your throat say if it could talk? Don't think! Don't try to make sense of all this! Just say what comes to mind! No censoring! Go!"

Now I hear a new message from deep inside. "I am not happy." Then a pause.

Ah, I think, the truth is coming out. The door of the body—and with it the unconsciousness—is opening. Her conscious mind is finally releasing its control. I begin to probe more.

"You are 'not happy' about what?"

"I am not happy with my husband anymore! We've been married for fifteen years. At the beginning, he was so romantic. He was taking me to dinners at nice restaurants; he was making wonderful love to me with romantic foreplay. Then we had our two kids and the romantic dinners and everything else that was lovely in our marriage disappeared. He started working longer and longer hours. He comes back late at night. Now, he even works all weekend. He doesn't spend any time with me and the kids. And as far as sex goes, he has no more time for foreplay. He just wants it late at night when he gets home, and now he only has time for 'quickies.' That doesn't work for me! I hate it. I feel used." Her voice breaks down and tears come to her eyes.

Here is the key to her symptom, the pain that has settled in her throat. What I've just heard is the deep origin of her illness. I am not surprised. Why? Simply because of the anguish and the intense emotion she is showing. A deep chord has been struck. She has just tapped into the emotional source of her agony.

Cynthia had been sitting on a volcano of anger with pressure mounting as, day after day, she endured the trials of an unhappy marriage. One way Cynthia kept her rage from erupting was to stifle her emotions. Part of her wanted to scream, and yet another part of her that wanted to save her marriage had restrained her voice and kept her from lashing out at her husband. This constant, unconscious tension inside her larynx stressed her throat, generating great pain.

So many of my patients come to me with similar stories originating with an unhappy relationship or marriage and accompanied as a consequence by bottled-up anger, frustration, and stress. They come to see me with what they initially do not realize are the symptoms of their unhappiness: perhaps throat pain, backache, stomach ache, or depression or many other possible symptoms. They don't understand that all these medical problems are really symptoms of the greater problems of their anger, emotional pain, and frustration. All because *their hot anger has nowhere to go but stay inside and burn them.*

Cynthia continues, "I am so unhappy, but I cannot tell him! I need to stay quiet, proper, and well-behaved like I was raised to be!" She stops talking, looking at me intently. I can see sadness in her eyes—or is it despair? She is waiting for my reaction.

Now, her controlling conscious mind is surfacing again. Here, the armor of self-protection is building up again and trying to distance her from her own anger and fear. That anger is being kept inside, a destructive force with nowhere to go.

Yes, people can be quiet, proper, and well-behaved, as their parents often teach them to be. That keeps society civil and peaceful. But what are they supposed to do when anger and frustration are fermenting inside of them? That is something that parents have never taught them because they had no clue!

Cynthia needs to understand and act upon this truth:

*Hot anger needs to be vented otherwise it burns its owner.*

"Okay, Cynthia, I get it!" I say in my most understanding voice. It is important that she knows I am on her side, welcoming, accepting, and not questioning what she is saying. Then, I add, "Let's use the pillows!"

She looks at me with a puzzled and curious expression on her face as I place six big pillows on my examination table and say, "Imagine these pillows are your husband. What does your throat want to tell him? You have permission to tell anything and everything that comes to mind. You even have permission to hit those pillows."

"Really?" she asks. Her eyes widen.

"Really!" I answer with a big smile, anticipating what I know from past experience will be an immediate, drastic change in her attitude and behavior.

"Are you sure?" she says with a malicious look in her eyes.

"I am sure!" I answer. I am the one curious now.

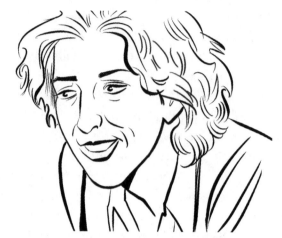

*Always ask in a gentle and welcoming way:*
*"What would my body say if it could talk? This could be*
*the answer of a lot of symptoms and illnesses."*

Then all of a sudden, her voice changes. It becomes spectacularly stronger as she continues talking and moving up close to the pillows.

"I am angry! I want to scream at you! I could hit you!"

We are on the right track. Now I push her while being supportive. "Go on, hit those pillows, Cynthia!"

She doesn't hesitate, hitting the pillows lightly, then with more force.

Not enough, I think. So I push her more. I want her to use more force to get a maximum amount of anger out of her body.

That's when she screams, "I hate you. I hate you. I hate you!" and she bangs on pillows harder and harder. Her outburst lasts almost five minutes.

"Oh it feels so good to let go!!!" she screams.

When her arms become tired, she says, "The pain in my throat is disappearing! This is amazing! How can this be, Dr. Chris?"

I explain to her that she has been experiencing anger and rage towards her husband for the last two years. With the pressure mounting day after day, a part of her wanted to scream at her

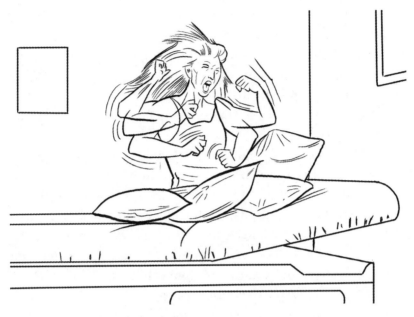

*Cynthia lets go: "I'm so angry at my husband!*
*I hate you! I hate you!! I hate you!!!"*

husband, to let loose and tell him how she felt. The other part of her, the polite, nicely raised girl, wanted to keep things together, not make a fuss, and not show any emotion.

It turns out that when we think of things we want to say, but don't say them, muscles in our larynx that control our vocal chords make small contractions as if we were speaking in a faint whisper. In Cynthia's case, these constant subliminal contractions associated with wanting to scream at her husband likely stressed out her muscles. And, as in all cases of voluntary movement, our vocal chords have two opposing sets of muscles: one set that moves our chords in one direction, and one that moves them in the opposite direction. Cynthia's urge to scream, and her equal desire to stifle her agony may have resulted in a struggle inside her larynx between two different sets of muscles. Both muscles may have become so tense that they were painful. This may explain her sensation of knots in her throat.

The other possibility is that the muscle layer of her esophagus was having spasms because of her stress. The only way to end this tug of war was to allow her to express her anger in a safe setting, under my guidance, against pillows.

"Wow, this was powerful! Thank you!"

And then she adds with a big smile on her face: "When can we do this again?"

I explain to Cynthia that she can do this on her own at home any time. I warn her to choose a time when she is alone, so no one can hear and she can be free of any restraints or self-consciousness. "Put a lot of pillows on your sofa and talk to them as if they were your husband. It will take the edge off and you will feel instantly better! Then, when your husband comes home, you will be less angry and you can ask him calmly to spend more romantic time with you like he used to do."

When Cynthia leaves my office, she is no longer the uptight, sad, pained person I saw just an hour earlier when she arrived. She is smiling, looking relaxed and beautiful.

Even to me, Cynthia's story sometimes seems too good to be true. How could a medical problem that persisted for months and resisted all conventional treatments, ease up after just a few minutes of releasing pent-up anger?

Science has found an answer. First, recent brain imaging research by UCLA neuroscientist Mathew Lieberman and colleagues has shown that the mere act of verbalizing negative emotions immediately decreases activation in a part of the limbic system ("emotional brain") called the amygdala. The amygdala plays a leading role in producing feelings of fear and anger. The common expressions "getting it off your chest," "letting off steam," and "venting" apparently have a strong basis in hard science. Exactly why simply verbalizing bottled-up emotions should be so immediately effective is unclear, but one strong possibility is that verbalizing taps into our unconscious, allowing emotions trapped there to escape.

This finding seems right to me. When we are thinking about something during a conversation, we don't know precisely *what* we are thinking (the exact words, for example), until we hear ourselves say it. It happens all the time. The formation of the exact words and phrases is the responsibility of unconscious parts of our brain, because speech is far too complex and occurs far too fast for our conscious mind to control each and every rapid movement of our vocal chords, tongue, lips, jaws, and breathing muscles.

This is why we are sometimes surprised by things that escape our lips. Our unconscious brain, given control, can verbalize "what it really feels" to vent its frustrations. My technique simply speeds up this process.

Even though I asked her to scream, an act that could actually have made her sore vocal chords worse, Cynthia found relief from her pain. We were now directly addressing the deep cause of her illness: her pent-up anger.

When we alleviate the deep cause of an illness we can produce rapid, deep cures.

This is the central idea of my practice, and of this book. Lasting cures, versus temporary symptomatic relief, come about *only when the root cause of disease is addressed,* and the root cause of disease is usually emotional.

In Cynthia's case, although her sore throat abated quickly, her marriage did not go from unhealthy to healthy overnight. But her reactions to the imperfect relationship did. She no longer remained quiet. Now, whenever she needed it, Cynthia knew she had a place to go where she could be alone and scream out her frustration while beating on cushions.

Eventually she was able to interact with her husband in a much calmer, more rational manner. She found the strength to confront him and talk to him about all the things that were upsetting her and hurting their relationship. I am happy to report that he listened to her and he heard her. He made the effort to spend

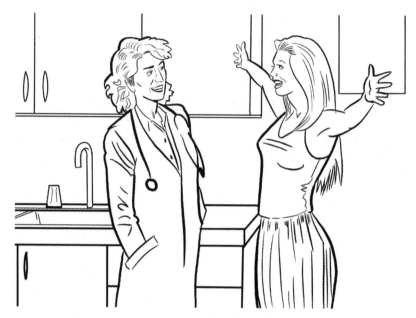

*After letting go, Cynthia is relieved,*
*and her chronic throat pain is much decreased.*
*"Thank you, Dr. Chris. I am feeling so much better!"*

more time with her, to try to be understanding, loving, and affectionate again. Over time, it worked. They are once again a happily married couple.

Cynthia's story is an important illustration of my methods and the reason why they work so well. The best way to explain it is that my patients are releasing pent-up feelings and stopping those feelings from damaging the body. We all know and have experienced what stress can do to us on a day-to-day basis when we encounter frustrating or unmanageable situations: We experience headaches, stomach aches, bowel problems, or panic attacks. Sometimes we even lose temporarily the ability to speak coherently—or to think rationally! If the situation causing our stress ends quickly, our symptoms generally will disappear just as quickly. But just imagine what happens if the situation is constant and unrelieved. That's when the real damage is done to our bodies, and that kind of damage is what I treat in my practice.

Cynthia's problem—and that of most people whose bodies suffer from stifled emotions—was that she was not consciously *aware* of the linkage between her troubled marriage and her suffering from the illness in her throat.

But Cynthia's body (specifically, her throat) was *very* aware of this connection, so by getting Cynthia's body to voice its anger and surface its inner conflicts, I led Cynthia to pinpoint the cause of her throat pain and to cure it.

So how could Cynthia's body be aware of the source of her problem while Cynthia herself was not? Put another way, how can a throat know things that the conscious mind, and Cynthia as the conscious human being, does not understand?

The key is the difference between the concepts of the "body" versus the "conscious mind." It is critically important to understand the difference in order to understand how and why my secret methods work.

This diagram, which shows the connection between Cynthia's body and her brain, along with memories stored in her brain, illustrates precisely what I mean by "Cynthia's body."

Each and every part of the body connects to a sensory part of the brain and a separate part of the brain right next to it that controls the body's movement (as shown in the diagram of the brain). Cynthia's throat and vocal chords, for instance, are controlled by her "motor" brain, while sensations from her throat and vocal chords are experienced in the nearby "sensory" part of the brain.

Each body part maps onto these two regions of Cynthia's brain, as shown in the drawing. Sensory input from Cynthia's vocal chords—such as sensations of vibration that accompany speech—cause a small group of vocal chord-sensory neurons to activate, making Cynthia consciously aware of throat vibrations.

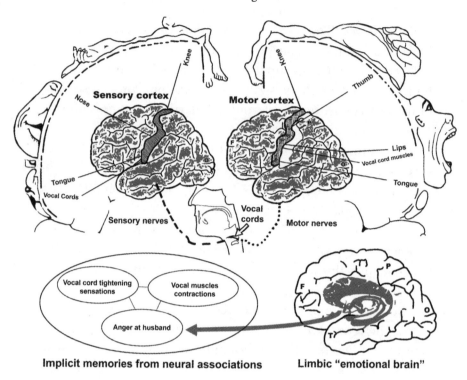

**Implicit memories from neural associations**     **Limbic "emotional brain"**

Conversely, neural excitation in a small region of nearby vocal chord motor neurons causes Cynthia's vocal chords to move. Notice that a completely separate set of sensory and motor neurons sense and control the tongue, the face, the hand, the back, arms, legs, and so forth.

The sensory and motor parts of Cynthia's brain also store memories of past sensory stimulation and movement, as do other regions of her cerebrum (which also store emotions during particular sensations and movements). These sensory and motor memories are almost entirely unconscious, because they contain vastly more data than Cynthia's conscious mind could process. As an example, think about how many tiny sensations and movements accompany each and every word that you say! As most people are likely to do, Cynthia suppressed her memories of anger because they could cause unpleasant fights with her husband.

Taken together, Cynthia's vocal chords, and the neurons in her brain that sense and control her vocal chords, constitute what I call "Cynthia's vocal chords," while the unconscious memories and emotions associated with her vocal chords are what I tap into when I give Cynthia's body a voice.

I gave Cynthia's body a voice by coaching her to become her throat, thereby shifting her identity into her unconscious "body" and memories, where the full knowledge of the link between her painful marriage and her painful throat resided.

You see, Cynthia's brain had observed that her vocal chords became stressed whenever she suppressed anger and the urge to scream: Cynthia just wasn't *aware* that her brain had observed and stored away this information. The formation of such unconscious memories of cause and effect among sensations, movements, and emotions is called implicit learning.

So, throughout the rest of this book, when I talk about giving the body a voice, I am not referring to abstract metaphors for the voice and the body, but concepts grounded in the neuroscience of emotion, implicit memory formation, perception, and movement.

How did I come to develop and use these unconventional ideas and techniques?

Well, let's go back in time. When I started practicing medicine thirty years ago, I thought I knew it all. I had people coming to my office "for the sensation of a lump" in their throat, stomach pain, back pain, fatigue, you name it. I was proud of the work I was doing: ordering tests, prescribing medications, and curing illnesses.

I was able to treat successfully a large number of patients. But for some, as with Cynthia, tests came back normal, but the patients would return to my office again and again, still complaining of their symptoms and, in addition, complaining of side effects of their medications.

I would then try to put them on different medicines, hoping that side effects would be more manageable.

As years went by, my pride diminished, and I became more humble, realizing that eighty percent of the people who came to see me had symptoms that were attributed to undiagnosed, untreated emotional stress. I came to realize this because, as a physician, I have been trained to think about cause and effect when evaluating possible reasons for a patient's illness. What had they eaten that would make them nauseous? Where had they traveled before they picked up an infection? What physical exertions preceded muscle pain? As I asked these questions, I noticed that patient after patient had emotional upsets or stress shortly before the onset of their symptoms. And symptoms often got worse when the patients' stress increased. As I pointed this out to patients, they often confirmed my suspicions. The conclusion was unmistakable: *The stress must be causing these symptoms.*

But what was I to prescribe then? Antianxiety drugs? I didn't like that option.

The drugs might work for a while but after a few months, they would become addictive because the amount of medication they were initially taking would become less and less effective. Increasingly higher doses would be required in order to produce the desired calming effect. Loading my patients up on these anti-anxiety drugs seemed to me to be the absolutely wrong thing to do.

I decided to try other modalities. I wanted to find out if other kinds of treatments were available to target the root causes of disease without side effects.

I studied homeopathy and acupuncture and used those techniques with success. They suppressed side effects, but often their action would only be temporary because they didn't reach the source of the diseases. What, then, would?

Since I didn't have the answers, I continued practicing conventional medicine, prescribing appropriate medications to people with serious infections, heart disease, diabetes, high blood pressure, and stroke or cancer survivors. I used homeopathy and acupuncture for symptoms that I believed were due to emotional stress. My approach worked well but not on everybody. I kept hoping I could find another way.

Eventually I did.

## A Healing-Secret Exercise

Let's try a practical exercise to help you give a voice to the area of your body that is showing symptoms of illness and link this to an emotion, and then to an action.

Sit down in a comfortable chair, close your eyes and take a few deep breaths.

Concentrate on your body.

Do you have any pain anywhere? Do you feel fatigued?

Do you feel sad or depressed?

How does your throat feel? Is it tense or relaxed? Are you experiencing any dryness, itching, or burning? There's no need to do anything at all except to just concentrate on this for a few minutes, and try to be aware of how it feels.

If you feel any pain anywhere, give your suffering body part a voice and have it link its pain to an emotion and then to an action.

For example, if you have pain in your lower back, start with "I am (your name) Sarah's lower back and I am in pain. I feel tense. I am linking this with anger or frustration or sadness or whatever comes to mind."

If you feel your pain is related to stress, anger, or frustration, go to a private soundproof place (an empty house or your car) and bring a few big plump pillows with you. There you can scream out your stress. Beat the pillows to vent out your anger or frustration. Cry out your pain.

You'll find that you will feel better immediately.

Use this technique any time you feel overwhelmed by feelings of sadness, anger, or frustration, or whatever other negative feeling you are experiencing.

# 2

# The Healing Secrets That Changed My Life

SOMETIMES WE FIND what we are looking for when we least expect it. That's what happened to me when I suddenly came across a scene that changed the way I practice medicine. I saw something that showed me how to treat patients and *heal* them instead of just treating their symptoms.

At the time it happened, about thirty years ago, I was living in France and practicing medicine there. I had taken a vacation to the United States and, with a friend, visited the Esalen Institute in Big Sur, California. Esalen is a well known retreat center and an educational institute devoted to new understandings of self and society. As we explored the place on the afternoon of our arrival, my friend suggested I attend an open seat Gestalt session. I had no idea what that was, but I was curious and so made an appointment for a session the next day. But much to my surprise, I was to experience Gestalt therapy much sooner than that.

Later that same afternoon, I casually and unknowingly walked into a room and stumbled upon a group of twenty people sitting on pillows in a large circle. They were all looking intently at one man also sitting on a pillow who was talking about how he felt trapped in his relationship with his longtime lover and live-in partner. The man looked like he was in his forties, with long brown hair gathered in a ponytail and brown eyes.

The session leader, sitting on a pillow next to the man, suddenly turned to him and asked, "Describe to me what it feels like to be trapped. What does your body feel here *at this exact second?*"

The man named Peter said, "I feel like I cannot breathe deeply. I can't get enough air into my lungs. It's as if I am suffocating."

I observed that something very important was happening.

Peter looked like he was having trouble breathing. Had we been in a hospital setting, I would have run to him, bringing him oxygen, and ordering him to lie down while I took his vitals. I suppressed my physician's impulse, as I was obviously just witnessing a session with the man who was leading a group. I needed to relax and trust that the leader knew what he was doing.

I didn't know it at that moment, but I later learned Peter was undergoing classic Gestalt therapy with his therapist who was coaching him to pit a conscious part of his psyche—which wanted to stay in the relationship—against another part that unconsciously wanted *out* of the relationship. Gestalt therapists believe that getting patients to "be in the moment" with strong feelings experienced by the different parts of their psyches brings hidden conflicts out into the open where the patient and therapist can deal with them. In a typical example of this kind of therapy, one part of the patient (perhaps the one they think of as "me") would address an empty chair representing an overly critical, judgmental parent that the patient has unconsciously internalized.

I had come into the middle of Peter's Gestalt session, just as the therapist was encouraging him to play the role of the part of him that felt trapped in the relationship

I was intensely curious to see where this would go. How would the leader handle the situation? My attention was glued to the scene.

Peter continued to talk, as he still appeared to have trouble drawing a breath. "This relationship is putting pressure on my body. It's like I'm in jail. There are walls around me, on me. I want to push them away! I want to be free!"

The facilitator seemed very calm and not worried at all. This surprised me. I was not feeling that way at all. Then he asked Peter to get up and asked for four volunteers to create "walls" around him with their bodies. Four men got up and surrounded Peter.

I was mesmerized.

Peter was tall and muscular. The men were equally well built.

The facilitator asked the men to press their hands gently against Peter's body. "Peter, is this giving you the same feeling of being trapped?"

Peter breathing hard, "Yes, this is exactly it."

The facilitator, after silently indicating to the men to increase their pressure, asked: "What exactly are you feeling now?"

Peter, while having more difficulty breathing and clearly struggling, said, "I feel pressure! Pressure on my heart, my lungs, my belly, on my back! I want to get out!!!"

The therapist silently again motioned the men around Peter to add more pressure and said aloud, "Peter, show us!"

My whole body was tense. My heart was in my throat. I thought this man was in danger of dying. I had to protect him. I was ready to shout, "Stop! I'm a doctor! You can't do that! This man is going to die if you press more! Can't you see? Stop pushing!"

But I remained, against my will, silent. My voice would not work. It was like I was hypnotized.

That is when the moment happened, the moment I will always remember, the moment that influenced the rest of my life.

Peter screamed, "I am trapped! I want out!!!"as he tried to push the men away, first using small force and a low voice, then using more and more force, struggling to break through, yelling at the top of his lungs, "OUT!!!!! OUT!!!! GET OFF ME!!!! GET OFF!!!!"

His screams were so loud that I reflexively covered my ears with my hands. Again, I did not intervene. It was a selfish decision, I admit. I was eager to know what was going to happen next.

The four men were putting more and more pressure on Peter, now using their whole bodies to press against him. As they were having a hard time keeping Peter inside their human wall, more men from the circle got up to help them. Some women also joined in. Peter was completely imprisoned by all the bodies, screaming his lungs out and using all his strength as he tried unsuccessfully to break out.

There was so much energy, so much strength inside of him that I was flabbergasted. After a few minutes of screaming and pushing—and what felt to me like an eternity—Peter got tired and stopped. The men and women walling him in took a step back.

The facilitator remained calm and in control. I guess he had seen this many times before. "Peter," he said, "what are you feeling in your body now?"

Peter, catching his breath and deeply inhaling and exhaling, said, "I feel relief!"

I was stunned by his words and even more by the way he looked. He was taking long, soothing deep breaths with his eyes closed.

The individuals who had made up his human wall took their places in the circle and sat down on their pillows. Everyone in the circle silently watched Peter.

After a few seconds, he opened his eyes and looked at the people around him, and speaking with a kind voice and grateful eyes said, "Thank you. I thank you all." He seemed serene—very tired but somehow balanced.

What the therapist had achieved was spectacular. I was in a state of awe.

As I was staring at Peter with wide open eyes, it suddenly hit me. That was a huge amount of energy that had been bottled up in Peter!

Were other people like him? Did my patients have as much pent-up energy trying to get out? Could trapped energy cause disease if it were not expressed and dealt with? Could Gestalt therapy cure the cause, not just the symptoms of disease without side effects?

In short, was Gestalt the "holy grail" treatment I had been looking for all these years?

One question had always haunted me: Why did some patients have terrible lower-back pain when their X-rays and MRIs were only slightly abnormal when other patients had drastically compressed discs and vertebrae without any pain at all? Was the pain indirectly due to chronic psychological and emotional stress and directly due to muscle spasms? *Were the kind of volatile emotions that had been bottled up in Peter the source of some patients' otherwise unexplainable back pain?*

Getting more excited, I reflected upon what I knew about scientific links between emotional stress and disease. For decades physicians had suspected that disorders such as stomach ulcers, colitis, psoriasis, and hypertension had emotional roots, and they had prescribed relaxation, a job change, and psychotherapy along with conventional medications.

Encouraged by suggestions in "orthodox" medicine of a relationship between bottled-up stress and disease, I grew more excited and intrigued by the idea of applying Gestalt as an unorthodox treatment of physical illness.

What if I could adapt the Gestalt principle of giving different parts of the psyche a voice to instead giving different parts of the *body* a voice? Just as mental pain, as I saw in Peter, can arise from conflicts between different parts of the self, perhaps physical pain can arise from conflicts between different parts of the *body* or the mind. I began to think, what if I could coach patients to play the role of an ailing body part versus the reasoning of their conscious mind? Maybe, just maybe, it would uncover the true source of the body's ailment.

As I thought about this idea, I grew more excited. While Gestalt therapists aim for emotional healing in their patients, I began to see emotional healing as a means to a different end: *healing the body*. Emotional healing, of course, would be a big bonus, but my true goal as a physician is to heal the body.

I began to try it on myself. One day I would concentrate on giving a voice to my lungs, by saying things like: "We feel like we are breathing fully today; each of our alveoli is expanding with each breath and deflating with each exhale."

Another day, I concentrated on my sense of taste and smell, giving those senses a voice: "The air tastes a little acidic. I can smell a little pollution. And I can smell the flowers sitting in a vase next to me."

I loved the exercise.

I decided to push the technique further and apply it to symptoms. When I got a belly ache, for example, I experimented with giving my poor stomach a voice: "I really wanted this chocolate cake, but now I have so many cramps! I am feeling the cake covering my cells with unhealthy sugar. The pleasure was not worth it! I won't have chocolate cake anymore."

Another time, when I got a feeling of painful tightness in my throat during a week spent with my mother-in-law, I gave my throat a voice: "I wish I didn't have to remain nice and polite! I wish I could tell my mother-in-law I disagree with her! I am so frustrated!"

Becoming the voice of these various parts of my body didn't always relieve the pain, but it taught me to understand these techniques better. I enjoyed discovering more about my body by giving it a voice.

From here I developed the first of my healing secrets: When faced with a patient's chronic pain, fatigue, or depression, expose the unconscious conflict and allow the patient to vent the repressed feelings. The venting can be achieved by encouraging the patient to scream or act out by hitting pillows or a punching bag so that feelings are safely directed outwards and not kept inside where they damage the patient's body.

I have found that taking such actions often allows me to prescribe lower doses of conventional medication to patients or even to end their use completely—thus avoiding the medications' often uncomfortable or dangerous side effects.

I began to use the technique myself to avoid taking antidepressant pills when my dear, late husband was dying of brain cancer.

Watching my husband fight with the little strength he had left while succumbing little by little, day after day, to his illness was so painful for me as to become unbearable.

Of course, he was the one who was sick and suffering. Yes, it was unbearable *for him,* but I should have been able to handle it. Yet it couldn't. I was his doctor, his nurse, his driver, his cook, his wife, his lover, and I was watching him slowly die. I found it almost impossible to carry on, to refrain from crying in front of him, to force myself to seem the cheerful person he was used to living with.

I became very tired and depressed. So much sadness! So much frustration! So much anger! I had so many feelings bottled up inside of me! I felt as though I were full of molten lava burning up my insides, lava that might burst through my body at any moment.

I became more and more fatigued and despondent. My body and my mind were suffering.

Were prescription medications the answer? Should I see a physician to request antidepressants?

But I decided that I would refuse to go down that road and began looking for a better answer.

I applied my pillow technique: One morning, feeling particularly bad, I grabbed a few pillows, went to my car, and drove to a park and screamed and banged on the pillows for what seemed to be an eternity.

I screamed and railed against the universe, against brain cancer, against the unfairness of life.

The more I screamed and hit those poor pillows, the better I felt. When I came back home that day, I felt much less depressed and exhausted despite the intense physical exertion. I found that taking care of my husband seemed easier.

During the next year and a half of his illness, I went to my secret place almost every day, liberating as much emotional pain as I could by yelling, screaming, and hitting my pillows.

This allowed me to remain sane without resorting to drugs for anxiety and depression. This is what allowed me to live with the unbearable while continuing to work in my private medical practice.

Later on, a patient came to mind who I thought might benefit from working with pillows the way I had. She, too, was taking care of her husband who was dying of pancreatic cancer. She, too, was very tired and depressed and was experiencing back pain. Side effects from pain medications became so severe that she chose to endure her pain rather than take the analgesics. I was treating her with homeopathy and acupuncture, but she still had a low level of back pain. I asked if she was willing to try something new. When she agreed, I tried my new technique on her. She loved it and felt immediate lessening of her pain.

Through my experiences I learned that people's unconscious struggles can manifest themselves in many different ways in their bodies. As we saw in the last chapter, Cynthia's inner struggle gave her throat pain with the sensation of a lump. Mine caused fatigue and depression. Others will have stomach pain or headaches.

A significant advance in the development of my healing secrets came when I discovered that a very frequent body target of these unconscious struggles is the back—both the upper back and the lower back. This is an interesting finding, considering that back pain is the second leading cause of visits to primary care doctors and will affect about eighty percent of people during their lifetimes. I began to wonder how many of these cases of having a "bad back" are due to undiagnosed stress rather than from some physical cause.

Some medical research suggests that emotional distress and repressed feelings, particularly rage, are responsible for the majority of back pain cases! It is claimed that when stress hormones such as adrenaline are released, they cause blood vessels to constrict in soft tissues of the back, including muscles. The reduced blood flow through the narrowed vessels starves tissues of oxygen and contributes to a buildup of metabolic waste products that promote back muscle spasms. Plus, adrenaline directly excites muscles of the back, making them more likely to sustain tension and develop spasms. Other studies have shown that hormones such as cortisol that are elevated in patients with chronic stress inhibit healing.

One of my patients suffering from chronic lower back pain was a forty-one-year-old man named Jackson who was working long hours for a very demanding boss in a law firm. By giving voice to his lower back, we uncovered that it was carrying a heavy load that was not as much physical as it was emotional. It was all too much for him.

During treatment, I learned that his work and his commute required Jackson to remain in a seated position for eight to ten hours a day. Adding to immobility, his frustration and anger were so intense that his paravertebral muscles (muscles on each side of his spine) were constantly tensing up, and this caused intense chronic pain.

How did Jackson's pain start? There was no physical trauma. He didn't fall or play a violent sport, and yet his pain was intense. Could an unacknowledged inner conflict be triggering his pain?

When he came to see me, his back was so stiff he could hardly move.

Under my guidance, Jackson began punching the air. During this exercise, he gave voice to his painful back in a conversation that revealed the true source of his medical condition—a conflict

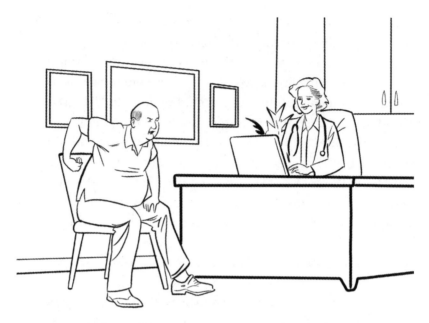

*Jackson: "My back hurts so much, Doctor Chris!"*

between his desire to support his family and the dreadful three hour commute to and from his unsatisfying job in an unreliable car that was constantly breaking down.

Like most people, he was not aware of the war being waged in his mind and body, but his hidden anger and frustration were showing up as extreme lower back pain. Jackson actually hated his job and was angry at having to waste three hours commuting every day. His mind dismissed these urgent messages, causing his lower back to "shout" ever louder by getting stiffer.

We began his cure by giving voice to his pained muscles which revealed the inner conflicts plaguing him. But there was more to do. He didn't beat up pillows in my office, but the answer to his problem was similar.

I instructed him to get a punching ball at home and vent the anger and frustration with a combination of screaming and hitting the ball every evening as soon as he got back from his office.

When Jackson came back to my office for a follow-up visit, I asked him to stand up in front of me and stretch his back to the left, to the right, bending over and bending backwards.

He looked reluctant, as if expecting pain, but as his back started to stretch out, his expression radically changed from frowning with anxiety to glowing with pleasure. "Ah this feels so good, Doc," he announced, stretching more and more, again to the left, again to the right, and backward and forward.

He was discovering something new, and he was in awe of the procedure and its effect. I was amazed at his body's reaction. He couldn't stop stretching. When he stopped for a few seconds, it seemed as though his back wanted more, and he would begin stretching again. His expression was pure delight, as if his back had been in a cast for several months and suddenly, with the cast gone, he was rediscovering what it was to be able to be flexible again.

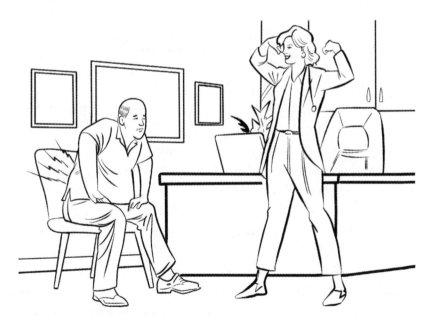

*Doctor Chris: "I invite you to do just like me.*
*A little stretching can go a long way."*

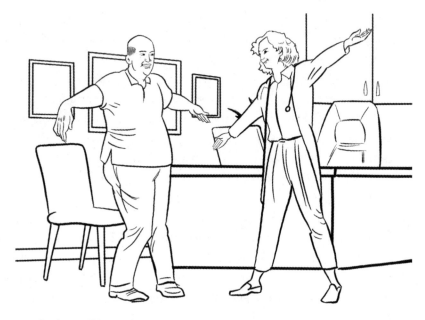

*Jackson: "I haven't done this in years, Doc! That feels really good!"*

I asked, "When is the last time you stretched your back, Jackson?"

Jackson continuing to stretch, looked surprised and responded, "Oh my God, Doc, I don't remember. It's probably been a really long time."

Looking at the way he and his body were reacting, I knew we had found the missing element for his complete healing: regular stretching exercises.

In Jackson's case, to solve his immobility problem, we decided to have him get up from his desk every hour and a half to stretch his back. He followed my instructions and the stiffness progressively melted away.

Jackson did not have to change his life. His pain problem was controlled through releasing his anger through action—punching that ball and stretching. It is so often true that cures require drastic lifestyle changes and thus ultimately fail because they are

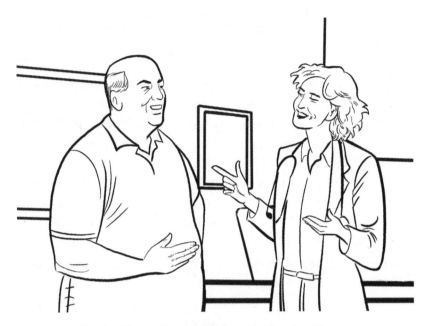

*Doctor Chris: "If you stretch every couple of hours,*
*your back pain will decrease.*
*It's never good for the back to remain sitting at a desk*
*6 to 8 hours a day without moving around."*

too much work. Happily for Jackson, physical action alone did the trick.

A lot of people are in Jackson's situation, having to sit for long hours at a desk without moving. They suffer from backache and also leg cramps. Because of gravity and muscle tension, their vertebrae are pushed against each other, squeezing the cartilaginous discs that are separating them. Blood tends to accumulate in their lower legs since immobile muscles are not pumping blood back towards the heart. Ultimately, their back and legs will let them know that they need to move to get the blood flowing freely. Since they can't talk to their owner directly, the only way for them to request movements is through pain. Only then will their owner pay attention to them. Their backs will have muscle spasms, and their legs will have cramps. What most doctors do in this case is to prescribe medications. But the real question to ask is, "*Why* does my back have muscle spasms; *why* do my legs have cramps? Are they trying to tell me something? How can I decipher their message?"

These are the questions I try to uncover with my unconventional way of looking at symptoms. I tried my techniques on countless patients. Cynthia, discussed in the previous chapter, and Jackson, discussed in this chapter are two of the many people I have helped.

There was only one problem: My new form of therapy often required me to devote at least one hour in face-to-face meetings with my patients. They loved the technique, loved to have their bodies talk, and loved to have mind-body conversations. But would their medical insurances pay for the extra time beyond what time was allotted for reimbursement? Some of the companies did. Others did not. But money wasn't that important to me. I cared and continue to care more about quality of life issues. My quality of life was improved greatly through the satisfaction I felt in helping people when other medical professionals couldn't. And of course so were my patients' lives.

My resolve to continue developing and practicing as an unconventional doctor was hardened by my medical past. I had traveled all over the world, had worked with Doctors Without Borders in refugee camps in Africa and Asia, and I had experienced many illnesses that required aggressive conventional treatments. But I had also seen so many ailments and symptoms in every part of the world that I was convinced were due to emotional problems. Why were all these sufferers being prescribed medications when other healing techniques were available? Why expose our patients to drug side effects and medication mistakes?

Pharmacists can mistakenly dispense one medication instead of another that sounds similar or is written in a similar way. For example, if instead of giving a patient hydroxyzine (anti-itch medication), they mistakenly understand and give out hydralazine (prescribed for high blood pressure), the patient could have a sudden drop in blood pressure, faint, fall, hit his head, and die. Physicians and pharmacists could make a mistake in medication dosage that, instead of curing, will kill. Why expose patients to such risks if they can be avoided completely?

And why needlessly expose patients to surgery (in people suffering from lower-back pain for example), if the correct diagnosis is emotional suffering or stress?

In the USA alone, 1.3 million people are injured every year from medical mistakes associated with misdiagnosis or drugs or surgery. And 400,000 people per year die because of these medical mistakes. Did you know that medical mistakes, if we were taking them into account, would be the third leading cause of death in America?

So I continue to provide my patients with ways to become aware of their bodies. I continue to ask them to be aware of what their bodies are feeling. I continue to show them that by giving their bodies a voice, by expressing their frustration and anger, or giving the body the movement and stretches it needs, they can rid themselves of stress, of inner conflicts, and the resulting symptoms of illness—usually with little or no medication. And, as you will see throughout the course of this book, I have developed a number of unique and unusual ways of finding the emotional source of illness, investigations that need to take place before I can begin to treat my patients.

These methods minimize the chances of medical mistakes from misdiagnosis by getting to the true root cause of illness. My techniques also reduce other types of medical errors by greatly reducing the use of drugs or surgery.

My journey continues since that wonderful day at Esalen, and my goal continues to be finding the best and most effective ways to heal my patients and to never be bound by the confines of traditional medical practice.

## A Healing-Secret Exercise

Let's try an exercise to discover how your body feels and what movement feels good.

Sit down in a comfortable chair, close your eyes and take a few deep breaths.

Concentrate on your body.

How does it feel?

How does your upper back feel? How does your lower back feel? Are they tense or relaxed? Do you have discomfort anywhere? How do your arms and legs feel?

Try stretching your back, your legs, your toes, your arms, your fingers. How does that feel? What movement feels good? What doesn't?

Remember what movements feel delightfully good. When is the last time you did those?

If it is a long time ago, try to incorporate those stretches in a routine every day, when you wake up and when you take work breaks.

# 3

# Connecting with Our Gut Feelings

A NEW PATIENT ARRIVES in my office one morning. She has come to discuss her weight gain.

I am truly impressed by her size. Amanda is severely obese. She is having trouble walking, and she appears short of breath after only a few steps into my examination room. She is wearing an extra, extra large, short-sleeve, baggy, dark brown dress that stops at mid-thigh, white flip-flop shoes, and no jewelry other than a black necklace.

I greet her, and she responds in a soft, polite voice that is in sharp contrast to her huge body and awkward appearance.

She glances at the armchair that I've routinely motioned her to sit in, and an embarrassed look comes over her. I follow her gaze and blush.

There is no way she is going to be able to sit on that narrow armchair.

I apologize, go to the waiting room, and grab a big, sturdy chair for her.

With a hesitant smile, she carefully positions her body above the center of the chair before slowly sitting down, legs open, with part of her bottom hanging symmetrically on either side without any chair support. Clearly, she has encountered this difficulty with chairs before.

She is the heaviest woman I have ever examined in my office.
Her belly hangs down to her thighs. I notice her legs and feet are
swollen and that could mean heart or kidney problems or bad
blood circulation in her legs. This woman is in trouble.

I try to evaluate her weight and estimate that she is probably
close to 400 lbs. It suddenly hits me that I won't be able to weigh
her accurately because my scale doesn't go over 350 lbs. That is a
problem. I should have bought a better scale. How will I be able
to monitor her? Maybe another physician in the building has a
more appropriate scale that I could borrow.

Confident I will find a way to weigh her, my thoughts go back
to the chair Amanda is sitting on. For a few seconds I worry that
it will collapse under her weight.

My concern must show on my face because I hear her say,
"Don't worry Dr. Chris, your chair is perfect." She has guessed my
thoughts and has a smile on her face.

Amanda is pretty with her long blond hair, a small turned up
nose and bright blue eyes. What happened to her? How did she
get so obese? I look at the questionnaire she has filled up while
in the waiting room: Amanda is twenty-five years old, only five
feet one inch tall, and weighs 373 lbs. Hmmm, I was right. She is
too heavy for my scale. But I can't worry about this now. I need to
focus on her.

"How can I help you, Amanda?"

Amanda replies, "Dr. Chris, I am tired of being so heavy. I am
tired of trying different diets. None of them work for very long. I
want to find something that will really work for me."

I realize that she apparently means my way of giving the body
a voice to reveal the inner source of ailments. I see on the form
she filled out she has been referred by another patient of mine
who had great success in losing weight, so she may have heard of
my unorthodox techniques.

In my practice, I have found that it is vitally important to focus
on what the body is feeling and to try to give it a voice to make it
a part of our conscious understanding. As I described in chapter

one, allowing the body to then act out by yelling, screaming, and punching (pillows), or as shown in chapter two by engaging in other physical action like stretching movements can affect an emotional catharsis by allowing stress and pressure to escape from a suffering patient and help to alleviate symptoms. My sense of Amanda is that this kind of exercise treatment is not what she needs.

Sometimes I've had good success with another method of encouraging my patients to create monologues or dialogues involving parts of their bodies—in this way finding the "voice" of relevant organs or areas of their bodies—as well as the voice of their conscious minds.

First we will explore the case of Amanda who will benefit from giving her stomach a voice in order to find the deep origin of her overeating. Then you'll meet Patricia who is also overweight, but we get at the source of her problem through a different means: finding ways to bring out in the open the conflict between her mind and her body. Finally, Eve will directly tune into her body's feelings to find the origin of her intensely bloated and painful abdomen.

I find that often when patients complain of pain, I can quickly zero in on the hidden source of their ailments. I am wondering if that will be the case with Amanda. Does she have any pain? Recalling her shortness of breath after just a few steps, plus her swollen legs, I think she probably does have pain somewhere. So I ask her.

Her response is not a surprise.

"My belly hurts."

Ah, she does have pain! So I am on the right track. I now feel confident that my methods will work. But I wonder what we will find when I ask her to let her body speak. The belly is the obvious place to start given Amanda's pain location.

I watch her face carefully as I say, "Let's pretend that your belly can talk, that it can say whatever it wants, whatever it feels. What would your belly say right now?"

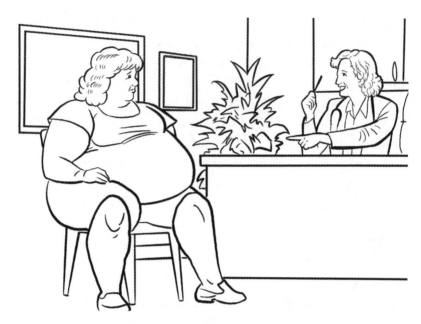

*Doctor Chris: "If your stomach had a voice, what would it say?"*

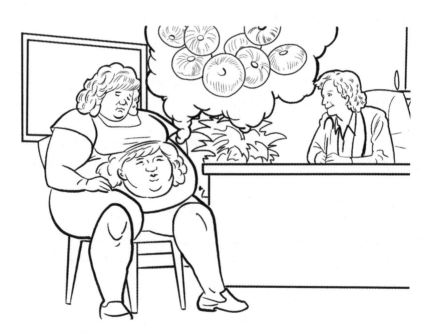

*Stomach: "I am constantly hungry! I love donuts!
I crave donuts! I dream of donuts all the time!"*

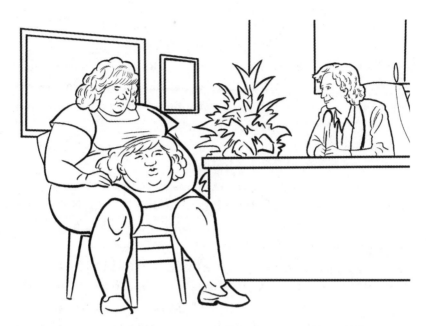

*Doctor Chris: "Why are you constantly hungry, Stomach? Is anything frustrating you?"*

She looks confused—not an unusual reaction with my first-time patients. "Ehhhhh. I don't understand. What do you mean?"

"I know it seems strange, but I just want you to relax, open up, and say out loud whatever your belly could say if it had a voice. Perhaps it will be easier if you start by describing your belly. Give that a try."

Amanda still seems puzzled by my request, but she looks at her very large and drooping belly with curiosity, almost as though she is looking at it for the first time "It is very big. It is hanging out. It isn't pretty."

"Okay, now switch it around and talk as if you *are* your belly. Like this, 'I am big! I am hanging out'. . . . Continue, please!"

Amanda looks embarrassed, but a shy, soft little voice emerges: "I used to be small and cute but now, I am huge and ugly. Amanda can't look at me in the mirror anymore. Now not only am I ugly, but I am hurting."

"Where is your pain?" I ask.

Amanda points to her upper belly. "There."

"Okay, that's where your stomach is located. It's the organ where the food you eat collects as the digestion process starts. Let's switch and focus on your stomach. Give your stomach a voice. What does it want to say?"

Amanda takes a moment to reflect and then says, "I have too much food inside of me. It's hurting me."

I am glad that Amanda's Stomach is aware that it is eating too much. This is a good beginning to be sure. Some of my over-weight patients aren't at all mindful of their eating habits and their overconsumption of food.

Now, my mission is to find out why Amanda is putting so much food in her stomach. Addressing her stomach directly, I ask, "Amanda's Stomach, what are you feeling?"

Giving voice to her stomach, Amanda replies, "I'm feeling empty. I'm hungry all the time."

"Any idea why you're hungry all the time?"

The stomach is "speaking" freely now. "Amanda is so big. She needs a lot of calories to survive!"

"What if Amanda didn't need all those calories? Tell me an-other reason, Stomach, why you want food all the time."

The voice remains silent for a while. Then with a big laugh, it exclaims, "Because I'm a food addict! Food tastes so good, espe-cially donuts and, above all, cheesecake! Hmmm!" Amanda is looking at me with mischievous eyes. I almost feel that I am star-ing into the eyes of her stomach, if such a thing were possible.

I smile at her. "Tell me, what do you feel when you are done eating your cheesecake?"

After a few seconds pause, the voice responds, "Then I crave more of it."

"So tell me what happens if there is no more cheesecake and no more of any kind of sweet food left to eat."

A serious look washes over her face. "If there is nothing more around me that I can eat, I feel really bad."

"How bad?" I ask, and Amanda's face changes. Now she looks very worried. My attention is drawn to her fingers, and I notice that they seem to have a tremor in them. "Really bad!" she replies. "I feel very anxious and restless!" She pauses.

I decide to wait. I am watching her body. Her eyes are frowning. She is biting her upper lip. The tremors in her fingers are increasing. All this is happening without Amanda being aware of this. What I am seeing is a reflection of her unconscious. There is turmoil inside. I remain silent, letting the process happen in a spontaneous way.

Now she is almost whispering, but I manage to hear that small voice again, "Amanda could lose control!" She is looking at me with apprehension. She seems frightened.

Ah, this is the moment I have been waiting for. The link between overeating and deep-seated emotional strife, in this case, fear of losing control, is out in the open.

Amanda's stomach knows that if it doesn't have food in it at all times, Amanda gets very anxious and she could "lose control" of herself. Amanda herself needs to learn this.

Now I need to find out what actually would happen if Amanda should ever lose control. The key to her overeating is sure to be in the answer to that question. How can I ask in a non-threatening way? My way is to ask the question not directly to Amanda herself but indirectly to her stomach, which, in my practice, becomes the door to her unconscious.

"Amanda's Stomach," I ask, "What is the worst that could happen if Amanda loses control?"

Will Amanda's Stomach reveal Amanda's deep issue? I am holding my breath.

Tears come to Amanda's eyes. That means, in my experience, that the deeper issue is about to come out. I am eager to know but decide to wait patiently.

"*If Amanda lost control, she would leave Gregory, leave Ethan, leave everything.*" A river of tears comes to her eyes.

This is it! This is the core of the problem! The intensity of Amanda's emotion makes me believe that we are getting to the source of her problem. We are seldom aware of the deep emotions that drive our behavior. Our lack of awareness can keep our negative emotions bottled up inside where they can damage the body.

In Amanda's case the corrosive, bottled-up feeling is helplessness. Gregory controls her life, her overeating controls her life, and now her *obesity* controls her life. In short, everything but Amanda controls her life. She is helpless. Such overwhelming helplessness in the face of adversity is perhaps the single biggest source of chronic stress—and stress-induced illness—that I see in my practice.

The first step in dealing with helplessness is to get a patient to become fully *aware* of the depth of their feelings of helplessness, so that they can understand the importance of taking even small steps towards taking back control of their life.

With this in mind, I decide to probe deeper while Amanda's guard is down and I can perhaps access her unconscious. "Stomach, what is the problem with Gregory and Ethan?"

Amanda hesitates. I hold my breath hoping she will continue to open up. She does. "Gregory runs everywhere for hours at a time. He is only five years old, but he is already strong and so energetic. Taking care of him 24/7 is so hard! And Amanda needs to do this for the next ten years, maybe even longer . . ." She stops talking and begins sobbing.

I continue with some gentle questioning. "Well, in ten years, he will probably not need your care 24/7 anymore! But let me see if I understand you, Stomach, you're craving all kinds of sweet foods all the time; I am guessing it isn't because Amanda needs calories, but then why?"

"Because it numbs the pain—the pain of Amanda's anxiety."

Ah, now, we have a relationship between food and anxiety. Amanda is eating to decrease her anxiety. I remember that research done at Harvard University suggests that eating fatty, sweet foods introduces substances into the bloodstream that temporarily inhibit parts of the brain that create feelings of stress and that trigger release of stress hormones such as cortisol and adrenaline. Studies have also shown that over sixty percent of overeaters suffer from anxiety, and for many, food simply becomes their "drug of choice."

I realize that food is Amanda's "drug" for suppressing anxiety and stress, but it's much more important that Amanda come to this conclusion on her own. That way she will be more motivated to act on her insight. I begin the process of getting Amanda to own the idea of food as a drug by asking a question.

"Ah, so food is like an anesthetic; is that right?"

Amanda suddenly realizes what is really happening and looks horrified. "Yes, that's right! Wow! That sounds horrible."

There we are touching another problem. People tend to judge themselves negatively if they don't do the things they think they *should* do. Yet what really matters is what *is*, not what *should be*. I need to reassure her.

"That is not horrible! It just is! What matters is what *is* real. There is no good or bad! No horrible or beautiful. There is only what is true today, here and now. This is what's important so that we can get to the core of the problem."

I know that the core of the problem is not only her son, Gregory, but also her husband, Ethan, as her stomach revealed. Now that the problem with Gregory is in the open, I need to find out what the problem with Ethan is. The way to do this is again indirectly, in a non-threatening way, by asking her body to tell me, in the first person, everything it is feeling.

After half an hour Amanda's body has given me (and her) three deep insights.

Taking care of Gregory consumes all of her energy so that she is constantly fatigued and dispirited. She also has grown to resent that she got so little help from her husband, Ethan, in caring for Gregory, even though Ethan has a full-time job and is the breadwinner.

Because her son is a full-time occupation, she has almost no time to do the things in life she enjoys most, such as playing her guitar. Before Gregory was born, another thing she enjoyed was sex, but Gregory's birth put a big damper on her sex drive. Her simmering resentment of Ethan further inhibited her sex drive.

In fact, she used her obesity to push her husband away precisely so that she *wouldn't* have to have sex with him.

I can now understand how all of the factors conspire to create a vicious circle for Amanda of overwork in taking care of her son, stress, helplessness, pain from anxiety, overeating to numb her pain, obesity, avoidance of intimacy, loss of everyday enjoyment, added stress, more helplessness, overeating, and so on.

Many doctors don't address those vicious circles and only tell patients to start a diet and physical exercise.

I didn't take this route with Amanda for two reasons.

First, patients rarely comply, over the long haul, with doctors' prescriptions for diet and exercise. Dr. Stephen Rollnick and colleagues at Cardiff University in the UK conducted behavioral research showing that when physicians instruct or direct patients to diet, exercise, or stop smoking, it rarely works. But when doctors simply lay out information about the effect of behavior on health and allow patients to reach their own conclusions, patients are much more likely to alter their behavior in healthy ways.

Second, diet and exercise, in any case, will only treat the superficial symptoms of Amanda's problem, not its deep emotional causes. Amanda is getting far too much anxiety relief from overeating and far too many free passes on sex to give up her "drug of choice," her food, so easily.

I have to find some way for Amanda to reach her own conclusions about a reason to change her deeply entrenched eating behavior.

I decide to probe for solutions first telling Amanda what I want to do next. "Let's ask your body and your mind what the solutions are!" Then I begin, "Stomach, what do you see as a solution?"

Amanda pauses before giving her stomach a voice. The voice that comes out of her sounds very strong, which is a sharp contrast with the weak voice Stomach had before. "There should be no more junk food in the house, only healthy fruits, salads, and vegetables."

"Thank you, Amanda's Stomach," I reply. Then to Amanda, "That sounds really good. I hear a big change in the voice. It is now much stronger than before. Did you notice that?"

"Yes, you're right. I didn't pay attention to that, but it is stronger." She smiles.

In all my years of practicing medicine, I have seen that I can learn a lot by paying attention to people's volume and tone of voice. Scientific research backs me up on this. Studies show that our tone of voice carries "honest communications" that are largely unconscious and signal our deepest feelings, particularly basic emotions such as anger, fear, disgust, sadness, and surprise.

Okay. It's time to move on and find out what Amanda is really thinking about these revelations. "Thank you, Amanda's Stomach! How about we now ask Amanda's Mind? Amanda's Mind: What do *you* think the solution is?"

Amanda pauses again before giving her mind a voice. Here too, the voice is strong and has a slightly lower-pitched tone than the previous two. "I am really happy having a beautiful son, but 24/7 is too much. I don't want to be a stay-at-home mom any more." She pauses, looking at me as if she is looking for an answer to an unspoken question.

Her lower-pitched voice tells me that what she just said is the deep truth that needs to be accepted, welcomed, and acted upon. It should not be dismissed because it may go against social norms or the idealized views of motherhood that the patient may have once held. I know that my goal here is to be supportive and to teach her how to find real solutions that will heal, not just to paper over the problems with superficial fixes.

I go on. "If you could do anything you wanted, what would you do?"

Amanda, her eyes gleaming with excitement, "I would love to go back to work as a waitress, go for walks along the beach, and play my guitar and sing again for fun."

For the first time in our session, I see hope in her eyes. For the first time, she seems really alive. We, as a team, are finding a possible long-lasting solution to her health problems.

I decide to mirror her excitement. "Great, perfect! Close your eyes and visualize playing your guitar and singing. What do you feel in your stomach?"

Amanda closes her eyes and murmurs, "I feel butterflies in my stomach."

Butterflies are a good sign, much better than pain. It is time to find a practical, realistic plan of action. "Realistically, who can take care of Gregory during your self time?"

Amanda reflects on this for the longest time. I can see she is struggling with the idea of somebody else taking care of Gregory. Her "shoulds" are still very strong like they are in a lot of people. I am patiently waiting. What is happening inside of her is so crystal clear. I am witnessing an internal fight between her body and her mind. Her eyes are frowning, her fingers are tight in a fist, her body is tightening. Finally her body relaxes, and she says, "I think I could pay for some daycare and ask my mother and mother-in-law to help babysit." Then looking thrilled, she adds, "They will be delighted!"

Her body has won. I am glad. "Perfect! Are all these ideas compatible?"

Amanda's eyes are beaming with excitement. "Yes! For sure!"

"Are they doable starting tomorrow?"

Amanda seems filled with energy as she answers, "Yes, I can even start tonight."

That is a great answer. The fact that she is truly enthusiastic and ready to start tonight means that these solutions are real for her. They will address her problems.

Amanda continues, "If I can go back to work and play my guitar, I won't need comfort food anymore. As far as eating, the friend who told me about you told me about your diet recommendations and why French people don't gain weight. I really like your ideas and your meal suggestions. It worked for her and she has made it her way of life. I want to try it."

(Please see "Dr. Chris's Diet" and "Why French People Don't Gain Weight" at the end of this chapter).

I am satisfied with her answer. I ask her to come back in one week. "Enjoy the first week of your new life!" I say as she leaves my office.

I see true happiness and excitement in her eyes.

When I see her the following week, she has lost her first ten lbs. She has substituted salads, fruits, and vegetables for fatty, salty, and sweet treats, has added probiotics to her diet, and is drinking water instead of soda.

A year and a half later, when I go to see her one evening at her house, she is hardly recognizable. She is gorgeous—170 pounds and still losing weight.

She has stopped working as a waitress and instead works as a health coach. She plays her music at night, which delights her husband and her son who is now six and a half.

With a smile, she takes me to her fridge. "Doc, can I offer you some lettuce, tomatoes, and cucumbers?" I look inside her fridge and am delighted to see that it is full of salad, vegetables, and fruits. We look at each other and burst out laughing.

This story of Amanda shows how by creating a conversation between the body (here, her stomach) and the mind, patients and I manage to uncover unconscious struggles that, once exposed, accepted, and even welcomed, allow patients to find their own long-term fixes.

Giving the body a voice to say directly what is going on with it works well with some obese patients. Other patients can benefit from a different approach where I encourage them to start a purely *internal* dialogue between different parts of themselves, rather than a direct dialogue with me. This technique, derived from Gestalt therapy's "empty chair" method, helps bypass psychological defense mechanisms that get in the way of self-awareness.

Gestalt therapy recognizes that we all have different facets to our personalities, such as selfish parts and caring parts, that often conflict which each other. When these conflicts cause emotional problems, such as feelings of guilt, Gestalt therapists ask a patient to imagine that one of their sub-personalities—say the selfish part—is another person, sitting in a empty chair across from them, and then have the other sub-personality confront the person openly. These confrontations bring deep, hidden, unconscious conflicts out into the open, increasing the patient's awareness of their inner struggle along with possible solutions for resolving the conflict.

Patricia is a good example of a patient whom I thought would benefit from such a vigorous internal dialogue.

Like Amanda, Patricia is overweight but her weight gain occurred only in the last five years. Up until the age of fifty-seven, she had been able to eat all she wanted without gaining weight.

During the last five years, however, despite eating the same high amount of carbohydrates and fats and exercising the same way, she has been gaining fifteen pounds a year for a total of over seventy-five pounds.

All conventional medical tests are normal, including her thyroid hormones level. They especially need to be checked when there is a weight problem in order to rule out a thyroid gland dysfunction. She is menopausal and her estradiol levels are low as expected at her age, but since she isn't experiencing hot flashes, she and her primary care physician have decided against hormonal replacement therapy.

When Patricia tells me that this is the first time in her life she's had a weight problem, I know exactly what the next step is. Patricia and her body are now sixty-two years old but her mind feels like she is thirty, and her behavior, especially her eating behavior, may still be that of a thirty-year-old. I have to make her aware that there is a deep disconnect in age between her body and her mind. The way to do that is to have them talk to each other.

I lead Patricia to my examination table. "Let's put your conscious mind, your conscious thoughts and feelings, on the side for now." I grab two pillows, one orange and one brown, from a corner of the room. I place the orange one at the foot of my examination table and the brown one in the middle of it, in front of Patricia. "Let's ask your body a few questions," I say, motioning her to sit on the brown pillow.

Whenever there are two different feelings inside of us, in Patricia's case one in her mind and one in her body, both compete against each other. Invariably, the stronger one shuts off the weaker one, which is no longer able to express itself. The weaker one stays repressed inside the body, unable to give its opinion. This repression can cause medical symptoms and even illness.

For example, imagine your parents are coming to visit and stay in your home for two months, even though you all don't get along very well when you are together. If your mind orders you to host your parents in your home for two months and your body tells you this will be too long a visit because it's too tiring and too stressful for you, an unconscious fight will ensue. Your stronger mind may be overwhelming and silence your body and force it to be a good host. During those two months, it is very likely that your body will let you know that the stress of hosting your parents for this much time is too much for it, and it will become sick or be in pain in some way. My role as a physician is to show you that this is happening.

Pillows of different colors, placed apart from each other, can be powerful tools for uncovering the conflicts. The pillows help patients get outside of themselves and begin identifying with a specific part of the body. I hope the technique will allow Patricia to give her conscious mind and her body full and equal voices.

"Patricia," I say, "let's pretend that this pillow is your body disconnected from your mind. It is only your body that we want to hear from. Patricia's Body: You heard Patricia's mind saying it doesn't understand why you're gaining weight when you're being fed the same things as what you've always been fed? Body, do you have an answer to that mystery?"

Patricia laughs, and, giving her body a voice, answers, "Not really."

Giving her a serious look, I say, "OK, I take it that you don't really know, but if you knew, what would you say? What has changed?"

Patricia's body reflects and says, "Hmmm, I'm getting older."

"What's happening to you as you're getting older, Body?"

Patricia's body answers, along with a laugh from Patricia, "I don't move as much."

Now we are on to something. With her mind out of the way, Patricia can be in contact with her body's reality. I need to probe deeper. "I understand that you, Body, used to move much more. What did you do then that you are not doing anymore?"

Patricia's Body is suddenly serious. "I used to play tennis twice a week, go to the gym twice a week and walk fast everywhere. Now, I don't play tennis anymore, I still go to the gym twice a week but I don't walk fast everywhere anymore. My pace is slower. Also my routine at the gym is less strenuous."

As she speaks, her back hunches over, and her eyes become dull. I make a mental note of this and say, "That sounds like a big change in burning calories. So, Body, do you think you need as many calories now?"

Patricia's Body doesn't hesitate. "No, I definitely need fewer calories."

"Thank you, Body," I respond.

That is the answer I need. What is unique here is that her body itself is bringing to her awareness that it needs fewer calories. It is now time to shift her attention to her mind. For that shift to be effective, I like it to be palpably visible. I ask her to get off the brown pillow representing her body and sit on the orange pillow representing her mind. Then, she can feel the shift and can be 100 percent her mind.

Interestingly, I notice that as Patricia makes the shift, her attitude changes. She is quick to get up from the brown pillow and sit on the orange one. Her back is now much straighter. Her eyes are brighter and wider. She actually seems much younger. The change is spectacular. She seems like a different person. That is the beauty of physically separating the body and the mind, by using pillows.

I begin a new conversation, now addressing Patricia's conscious, thinking mind. "Welcome, Patricia's Mind, how old are you?"

"Oh, I know I am sixty-two years old, but I feel like I am twenty years old."

"Mind," I say, "tell me more about yourself."

Patricia's Mind responds enthusiastically, "I have so many ideas, so much energy, I could run a marathon."

I am smiling. I can definitely see that. It is time for me to ask Patricia to come next to me and look at the two pillows from a third, neutral point of view so that she can find a fix to her real problem. "See Patricia," I say, showing her the orange pillow. "Your mind is young and is not aging. But your body," and I point to the brown pillow, "is aging, is moving less, is using far fewer calories. If you continue to feed it the way you always have, it will be overfed."

It is important to note once again that directed diets seldom work, so I engage in a back-and-forth with Patricia eliciting her ideas on how to reduce her food intake.

She finally concludes that her core problem is that her body can't burn off as many calories as when she was twenty. With this insight, Patricia hits on a simple, obvious solution: Serve herself smaller portions consistent with her "new normal" metabolism.

This is a good idea because aging does indeed change the body metabolism, and being aware of the changes can help us age gracefully.

Our metabolic rate steadily decreases with age, but our body's ability to regulate appetite and body weight also degrades with age, so that older people tend to put on weight. Unfortunately, weight gain actually accelerates the aging process. In studies on monkeys, restricting their calorie intake extended their lives. The same results have been found in studies conducted in every species studied from fruit flies to fish yeast to rats, so there is no reason to believe the same is not true for people.

It appears that the more we eat, the more "oxidative stress" we put on our organs, accelerating their decline. Another term for "oxidative stress" is "rust."

In other words, the more we eat the faster we rust out—literally!

That session, as simple as it was, changed Patricia's life. Her new awareness and understanding of her stage in life made her decide to decrease the amount of carbs and fat she was eating. The result was weight loss and energy gain.

In Patricia's and Amanda's cases, their symptoms were obesity. A final illustration of the health benefits of giving the body a voice focuses on another kind of digestive problem: abdominal pain.

When pain is the patient's complaint, I sometimes have to do more detective work, because the underlying problem is more likely to be physiological. (Although, as we shall later see, even purely "physiological problems" often have emotional roots.)

Playing a detective is one of the most enjoyable parts of my job as a physician. I get to immerse myself in a mystery, and match wits with Mother Nature. I particularly enjoy uncovering clues that are buried deep in a patient's memory that the patient *herself* is unaware of.

That's what I did in the case of Eve.

Eve looks like a very nice person when she comes to my office. She has a soft voice and smiles easily, which make me immediately like her. She has long, straight, dark brown hair which is loose and covers her shoulders, a red t-shirt, blue jeans and tennis shoes. She has just turned twenty-seven years old, weighs 115 lbs. and is five feet four inches tall.

She is coming to my office complaining of abdominal pain. She is working as an esthetician, and sometimes her abdominal spasms are so intense that she has to take breaks from her work. I ask her a few questions and learn that she has been experiencing stomach pain for the last six months.

I need to know if anything triggered that pain six months ago. Maybe she picked up a gastrointestinal bug, but six months is a long time for such a diagnosis. Bugs usually last a few days to a week, unless, perhaps the bug changed something in her immune system. The questions worth asking are "Did anything happen just before the pain started? Did you have indigestion?"

Eve thinks for a moment and responds, "No, I don't think so. Oh wait, something did happen but it had nothing to do with my belly. I had a cold that lasted about three weeks. Does that count?"

Ah, this might be the first clue. A cold six months ago means her body became infected by a virus or bacteria, which could have changed the way she is digesting certain foods.

I am getting excited. This is the detective stuff I love so much. Finding the first clue is always thrilling.

"Yes, it does count! This is actually our first clue! Let's find out more! For this, I need to examine your belly. Can you climb on my examination table and show me your belly?"

She complies, lifting her T-shirt off and unzipping her jeans so that her belly is exposed. I look at it and pay attention to the way it is breathing.

Eve is staring at me, wondering what I am looking at.

What I am looking at is the way her belly is moving. Not only do lungs move when breathing, bellies do to. They have a nice rhythm of pushing out when breathing in and pushing back in when breathing out. When people are severely in pain, that rhythm is not harmonious. But Eve's belly looks good.

My first impression is that there is nothing really life-threatening. She is too young for cancer. Maybe she has some food intolerance. That is the most likely explanation. The first thing that comes to my mind is lactose. Lactose intolerance gives abdominal pain and bloating in the whole abdomen. I need to check the location of her pain.

After warming up my hands by rubbing them against each other for a few seconds, I place them on Eve's belly without pressure. She looks very anxious, stares at my face, afraid of what my examination is going to reveal. She makes a little scream of apprehension but then relaxes. I wait until she is completely relaxed again, and then start pressing, exploring each part of her abdomen, each quadrant as we say in medical jargon.

"Ouch! Ouch!" she exclaims in a strong voice.

That voice indicates real pain. Indeed, I can feel a lot of swelling in her whole abdomen. Usually when it is in the right lower quadrant of the abdomen, I think appendicitis, when it is in the right upper quadrant, I think gallbladder problems, but here it is her whole abdomen. It fits the lactose intolerance theory.

I need to confirm that the swelling is due to gas. The way to do this is to transform the patient's body into a drum and to tap on it. In order not to hurt Eve, I place my right hand flat on her belly, the way I have been taught in medical school, and tap on my right fingers with the third finger of my left hand. My tapping resonates hollow. That is the undeniable sign of gas.

Eve sounds surprised, "Wow, that's loud!" Then, "Is it bad, Doc?"

I smile to mask my bewilderment. "No, Eve, don't worry, I'm sure it is a simple problem with an easy solution. We just need to find exactly what the problem is." The truth is that at the moment I am not ready to say why she is so bloated. Maybe it is something simple—maybe she's been eating beans?

As I have done with so many of my patients, I encourage her to "become" her stomach, and I ask her stomach questions looking for suspects, particularly those rich in complex carbohydrates (starches and sugars) that can be hard to digest in people who lack the right enzymes. When we don't properly digest these starches in the small intestine, they move to the large intestine where microbes ferment them, generating painful amounts of gas. Dairy products are another one of the usual suspects because many people, after they become adults, lose their ability to break down milk sugars called lactoses (thus, lactose intolerance), with the same result: fermentation and pain in the large intestine.

My questioning of Eve's stomach is unproductive at first, as I explore one dietary cause of her gas after another.

One after another, I rule out the common offenders: milk, cheese, beans, and various complex starches such as bread, pasta, and potatoes.

When I exhaust all the easy answers, I know I have to shift gears and sift through knowledge that Eve herself doesn't know she knows. As we'll see in a moment, our unconscious minds record our life events, especially significant events such as pain. That's why some detectives employ hypnotists to get at information that witnesses have unconsciously "recorded" but have forgotten how to access.

My sleuthing methods are somewhat more direct than hypnosis, but their goal is the same: surfacing important clues buried deep below the surface.

I explain my plan to Eve. "My theory is that bodies know what is good for them and what isn't. If you are eating something, and I suspect you are, that your body doesn't digest well, it probably doesn't really want you to eat it—whatever it is. So is it possible that you are forcing your body to eat something every day that your body doesn't really want to eat?"

This is an important question. I am asking Eve to listen to what her body is feeling when she is eating.

I have noticed that sometimes the body will be slightly nauseous or disgusted with a culprit food. For example, somebody who eats one bad oyster that gives them vomiting and diarrhea will be disgusted with oysters for a long time, just from being sick from that one bad oyster. Neuroscientists call this phenomenon "flavor toxicosis," which has evolved in our brain to protect us from dangerous food by making us feel nauseated when we even *just think about* a food we ingested right before getting sick.

Could Eve's body know what is making it sick? Could her body be reacting to the look and smell of a food that it "knows" will cause upset—even before Eve eats it?

I suspect she needs to do some homework, to write down what she is eating every day, write down what her body is feeling everyday, how much pain she is in after breakfast, lunch, and dinner, and come back for a follow-up appointment.

I am surprised when she answers, "Well, Doc, funny you're asking, I am forcing myself to eat a big salad for lunch and some lettuce for dinner because it's part of my diet to not gain weight, but my body really doesn't like that. I am kind of slightly nauseous when I look at my salad before I eat it. Does that help?"

I am in shock! Yes that helps! That's it! Her body has just given us the answer!

With a big smile I say, "Well, I think we have the answer to your problem!"

Eve's eyes widen. "I don't understand. What is it, Doc?"

Before telling her, I want to make sure I have the right diagnosis. "Would you say you're eating lettuce twice a day?"

Eve says, "Yes, I am." Suddenly realizing what I am saying, she looks at me with disbelief. "Do you think lettuce is making me sick?"

I nod. "I am not one hundred percent sure but, yes, it could very well be."

Eve shakes her head. "How can lettuce make anybody sick? I've never heard anything like this before!"

I explain. "Lettuce contains complex carbohydrates that some bowels don't have the enzymes to digest. That may be the case with you. If lettuce isn't digested properly, it will be taken up by gut bacteria in the large intestine and fermented into gas. There is only one way to be sure. Stop eating lettuce completely for one week, and call me at the end of that week."

Eve agrees.

One week later, she calls. "Doc, you were right! I have no more pain and no more gas! Lettuce was the culprit! Thank you so much!"

I am happy that she is healthy and well again.

Now, you, reader, don't get the wrong idea . . . I see it coming now . . . If you are on a diet, you are going to tell me, "Doc, that's why I hate salads! My body doesn't want me to eat lettuce. I am probably allergic to it. That means I can go back to my chips and salsa."

Not true!

You probably just don't like the taste of lettuce and miss all that tasty fat and sugar in your pre-diet foods. But if you have abdominal pain and severe bloating after eating a salad, then you might have a case, so you'd better go see your doctor.

The fact that the body knows what it cannot digest is called "implicit learning," where our brain unconsciously recognizes and stores away cause-effect connections. Psychologists used to think that we had to pay attention to events in order to store them away as memories, but recent discoveries have shown that our brains routinely learn associations and cause-effect relationships automatically, without us paying any conscious attention at all. For example, almost everyone can tell the difference between a fake smile and a genuine one because they've observed over and over again that people who "smile for the camera" look subtly different from people who laugh spontaneously at jokes. We may not know *why* we know a smile is fake, but we know for certain that it *is* fake because of implicit memories formed over a lifetime.

In the same way that we gain implicit knowledge about external events such as smiles, we form implicit memories about cause-effect relationships for *internal* events. We unconsciously register, for example, that our back muscles tighten up every time we get in the car to visit relatives who always argue with us. So, our back "knows" that our relatives drive it into spasms.

And Eve's brain had unconsciously connected the dots between eating lettuce and getting gas, so that when I asked her what her body didn't want to eat, her gut knew the answer, even though Eve herself *didn't*.

Eve's story shows that "gut feelings" are important. Our body stores information all the time whether we're conscious of this or unconscious.

The secret is to have access to this well of knowledge through bringing awareness to what our body feels and express this with words.


## A Healing-Secret Exercise

Concentrate on your stomach after you finish dinner.

What feeling do you have in your stomach?

If your stomach could express that feeling with words, what would it say?

Choose one sentence of your choice for example: "I feel too full," or "I should have eaten more vegetables or more salad or fruit," or "I am still hungry," or "I ate just right."

Write down your sentence.

The next day, before you start your dinner, read the sentence, then look at your dinner plate.

Is what's in the plate balanced? Are there plenty of fresh vegetables, fruits, and salads?

If yes, eat slowly and enjoy the taste of each different food.

Pause eating before you finish your plate of food and direct your awareness inwards. Check in with your stomach.

Did it have enough to eat already? Did it have too much? Does it want more? Make a mental note of what your stomach says.

Okay, now finish your dinner.

Then go back to the first line of this exercise: Concentrate on your stomach after your dinner.

What feeling do you have in your stomach, etc.

At the end of each dinner, repeat the exercise.

You will see that day after day, little by little, you will eat healthier foods with full awareness of what you are eating.

## Here's another Healing-Secret Exercise

PART ONE:

If you are at a party and are eating cake, concentrate on your stomach and also on your whole body.

How do they feel after eating a big piece of cake?

As you begin eating, everything might feel good, and you might even feel happy. But later, do things feel as good?

Usually they don't. Your body will feel tired and will be craving another piece of cake.

If you are not feeling too full or nauseous yet, have another piece of cake.

How do you feel after eating the second piece of cake?

Make a mental note of the feeling, then, if you are still not too full—or nauseous—yet, eat a third piece of cake.

How do you feel after eating the third piece of cake?

Is your body feeling good? Is your body feeling bad? Is your stomach bloated? Are you feeling tired?

Write that feeling down then go for a walk around the block.

How energetic are you?

Remember that feeling.

PART TWO:

Next time you go to a party, instead of eating cake, bite on delicious raw carrots, celery, snap peas, radishes, and cucumbers.

Then go for a walk around the block.

Write down how you are feeling and compare this to part one.

Chances are your body feels much better and much more energetic after eating raw vegetables rather than after eating three pieces of cake.

Try from now on to eat as few sweets as possible.

Enjoy eating fruits, salads, and vegetables; enjoy feeling energetic and healthy.

# Dr. Chris's Mother Earth Diet

**BREAKFAST**

*One fruit or one cup of berries*

*One cup of plain, unsweetened, fat-free yogurt*

*A handful of nuts*

*One cup of green tea or coffee*

**LUNCH**

*One or two large glasses of water to start the meal*

*A very large salad with as much as you wish of the following foods: lettuce (unless of course you have trouble digesting lettuce!), cucumbers, tomatoes, red peppers, orange and green peppers, mushrooms, radishes, celery, fresh parsley, fresh thyme, oregano, French tarragon, and raw carrots with olive oil and vinegar*

*One slice of French baguette*

**DINNER**

*One or two glasses of water to start the meal*

*Grilled chicken breast with rosemary and thyme surrounded by as much as you wish of steamed broccoli with fresh parsley, or*

*Grilled salmon with dill and lemon juice swimming in the middle of as much as you wish of steamed green beans with green onions and sliced almonds, or*

*Pork roast with fresh onions and garlic in a forest of as much as you wish of steamed cauliflower, carrots, and zucchini with rosemary, or*

*Grilled chicken breast with fresh ginger, which is great with as much as you wish of baby bok choy and shallots, or*

*Chicken breast cooked in the oven with red wine and as much as you wish of parsnips, turnips, and carrots.*

Notice that you can have as much salad and as many vegetables as you want and that the volume I tell you to eat is mostly water. This is key for losing weight—eating large volumes of low calorie food.

What you also need to know is that the more sweets you eat, the more sweets you will crave and the more tired you will become. The reverse is true: If you stop eating sweets, you will stop craving them, and you will feel wonderfully energetic and ready to take on the world.

Couple this advice with thirty to forty-five minutes a day of fast walking or any other type of physical exercise. Now you have a recipe for success.

## Why French People Don't Gain Weight

Have you ever wondered why French people eat four- and five-course meals and don't gain weight?

That seems so unfair, doesn't it?

Well, not really. Having been born and raised in France, I can give you six delicious reasons why the French don't gain weight.

**Reason #1:** The French go to farmers' markets where they buy fresh produce (rosemary, thyme, mint, oregano, parsley, fruits, salads, and vegetables) at least once a week.

**Reason #2:** French people cook. Going out to eat is very pricey in France and people cannot afford restaurants on an everyday basis. So, they cook, and since they love to eat, they use very delicious recipes.

**Reason #3:** They use very little salt and use a lot of aromatic herbs and spices. They cook with rosemary, thyme, oregano, parsley, dill, French tarragon, mint, cilantro, basil, etc.

**Reason #4:** They use very little sugar in their desserts, which allows them to taste the acidity of apples in apple pies and the bitterness of dark chocolate in chocolate cakes.

**Reason #5:** They take their time and eat slowly. The downside is that meals take forever and turn into a social event. But the upside is that it allows food to be chewed well and slowly digested.

Quickly gobbling up food makes us eat more calories because we don't allow our body's natural appetite control mechanisms to work properly. When food is broken down in our stomach and absorbed into our blood, our blood sugar rises, signaling a region of our brain called the hypothalamus to reduce our desire for food. But this feedback control on appetite takes time because conversion of food into blood sugar takes time. So when we eat quickly, we short circuit our appetite control, and our brains don't signal until much later that we are full. The result is that fast eaters consume more calories than slow eaters. And experiments have shown that slowing the intake of calories does really reduce total calorie consumption.

**Reason #6:** The French don't drink sodas. They prefer water and drink several brands of delicious flat waters like Vittel and Evian, or they drink sparkling waters like Perrier. Of course, they also have their glass of wine with dinner. And wine has been shown to have beneficial effects for some people!

# 4

# Sex Talk

THE HARDEST CONVERSATIONS I have with patients are often about topics that are the most important to their health. As we've seen in previous chapters, my patients had to be encouraged and coaxed to bring out the strong, repressed emotions such as rage and helplessness that were causing them serious medical problems.

Another critically important, but extraordinarily difficult topic for my patients, as well as for just about everyone else, is sex. While discussions that shine the light on good sex, or a lot of sex, are somewhat easier to talk about than other matters about sexuality, sexual dysfunction for most people is a taboo subject.

Although people generally understand that sex affects their emotional wellness, they seldom see how critically important it is to overall physical health. Sexual intimacy, of course, brings partners together, strengthens emotional bonds, and stimulates feelings of happiness, well-being, and satisfaction. In terms of the biology of sex, orgasms vent pent-up frustrations and tensions that can harm the body if not released, and they release oxytocin and endorphins (natural opiates) that relax us and elevate our mood. Orgasms also inhibit activity in the "fear center" of the brain, lowering our anxiety and production of stress hormones.

For these reasons, satisfying sex has been demonstrated to have these important health benefits:

* Decreased stress
* Strengthened immune response, including production of antibodies that fight infections
* Lowered risk of cardiovascular disease
* Lowered risk of prostate cancer (in men)
* Improved sleep
* Increased longevity
* Increased endorphin and oxytocin release, yielding happiness and sense of fulfillment

On the flip side, a lack of sex or unsatisfying sex is detrimental to health.

Sexless marriages are frequently troubled marriages, and troubled marriages are bad for health, particularly women's health. Marital stress can increase risk of heart disease, infection, and early death. Research has found that women in stressful marriages have more cardiovascular disease and inflammation than women in healthy relationships. This connection between bad relationships, ongoing unhappiness, and bad health happens because of chronic over-secretion of stress hormones that can result in a weakened immune system as well as sustained, higher than normal blood pressure and heart rate.

The bottom line is that sex really, really matters to your health. Since it is so important, I always ask patients about their sex life. Two hundred years ago, people were living only until forty years old, but now they live much longer. It is estimated that fifty percent of people born after the year 2000 will live to be at least one hundred years of age. That means you'd spend a lot of years with the same sexual partner if you were committed to having just one. If sexual dysfunctions exist in a long-term relationship, they should be addressed as soon as possible for the sake of the pursuit of good health and for the sake of the relationship.

So how does the curing of sexual ailments fit into my medical bag of healing secrets?

Earlier in the book, I showed how an emphasis on "letting out steam" by using physical actions such as screaming, beating on pillows, hitting a punching ball, or stretching can help get to the source of illness. I also introduced my technique of giving the body a voice through a monologue or creating a dialogue between the body and the mind. All those techniques involved working one-on-one with an individual patient. In this chapter, we will see that sometimes working only with the patient is not enough. In certain situations, in order to help my patient, I need to bring together patients and their partners. We give voices to both of their bodies, and we have conversations between the two bodies!

But as I mentioned, sex is one of those topics that couples don't want to talk about, especially if there is sexual dysfunction in their relationship. So I sidestep that problem by getting patients to shift their conscious identities from their normal everyday selves, where they are defensive and often in denial about strong emotions, to another less accessible, usually unconscious part of themselves where their defense mechanisms are much weaker.

My approach is related to Gestalt role-playing where participants are guided to shift their sense of self from "Me" to "Not Me." When we shift to "Not Me," we are able to leave behind the defense mechanisms and internal censors associated with who we think we are. When adopted successfully, the "Not Me" identity has *no* defense mechanisms that can hide away our feelings and desires.

I accomplish similar shifts by requesting that my patients make simple changes in the language they are using during our sessions. When patients change their first person "I" statements to represent something, like a body part that is not thought of as being "them," they automatically and unconsciously protect themselves from unpleasantness and conflict.

Here's an example of defense mechanisms at work. When I asked a female patient about her sex life, she said, "I feel OK about sex. I'm just too tired most of the time." It later became clear that she hated sex because it was painful and unsatisfying, but she didn't want to express all of her frustrations and pent-up anger over sex.

But when I am able to move my patient away from her "I" statements and into perhaps a body part that she would not normally consider to be "herself" the defenses melt away. Giving voice to her vagina, she might say, "I hurt when his penis penetrates me."

The technique is simple but powerful when it comes to sexual dysfunction. As in the example above, I have my patients shift their observations about themselves to their genitals, where "I" statements are much less threatening and feelings often come through uncensored. For this reason, genital "I" statements can be incredibly revealing about what people are really feeling sexually.

When working with couples, I will ask a man to give his penis a voice and a woman to give her clitoris and her vagina a voice. In this way, we can explore the truth of their sexual condition. Taboos about the subject and feelings of shame and guilt are avoided because the mind remains silent and protected. We can now freely hear what the uncensored penis, clitoris, and vagina think and want to say. We can now get straight into the heart of the problem, and from there, great solutions usually can be found.

I have seen so many sexually unhappy couples in my medical practice. Being a family doctor has enabled me to hear the wife's point of view during one office visit and the husband's point of view during another visit. Hearing them separately and openly talk about the other one has always been very enlightening. So often they have no clue about what the partner likes, dislikes, and expects in the bedroom. The usual pattern is that such couples drop completely any kind of sexual relationship, which increases their stress and depresses their immune system.

This is generally a very difficult situation to remedy, and the conventional medical practitioner approaches it by ignoring it completely. Most physicians do not view sexual frustration and pent-up anger as a cause of physical symptoms, and even if they did, they wouldn't feel qualified to provide sex counseling. *The most that primary-care doctors will do in such cases is to refer patients to sex counselors.*

I believe I have found a better way, and the rest of this chapter is devoted to my approach. We will meet two couples who are complaining of totally different symptoms. With one couple, it is frequent infections and depression; with the other, it's chronic back pain. As we will see, all these symptoms have one thing in common: an origin in sexual dysfunction. And in both cases, as we will see, I am able to find satisfying solutions that allow them to heal and get their health back.

Let's start with Chloe and Joe.

Because I am their family physician, I usually see Chloe and Joe, a married couple, separately. Chloe has frequent sore throats and sinus infections. Joe often comes down with the same symptoms a week or so later. Why do they have frequent infections? Are their immune systems compromised? For both of them, blood tests show no problems there. So the question, "Why are they sick so frequently?" remains a mystery for now.

One day, Chloe brings Joe to my office. He is just recovering from bronchitis and is feeling fatigued. Chloe isn't feeling so good herself. Both say they are always tired, not sleeping well, and not enjoying life very much. It sounds like they are depressed, which seems confirmed when they also explain they have lost interest in activities they once enjoyed, feel sad much of the time, and aren't thinking as clearly as they once did—all classical signs of depression.

Chloe is a twenty-three-year-old, short, slightly overweight brunette with hazel eyes and long hair that spreads across and over her shoulders, covering her large breasts. Joe is a handsome, tall, slim, twenty-six-year-old engineer with large, dark brown eyes.

When I ask questions about why they feel depressed, they can offer no apparent reason. Chloe is finishing her nursing degree and loves what she is doing. Joe enjoys his work as an engineer. They have a social network and apparently satisfying hobbies.

At their relatively young age, sex is usually important in a relationship. So, I decide to ask some questions about their sex life. They look embarrassed. After they exchange some awkward glances and nervous looks, Joe offers up their story:

They have no sex life.

As Joe tells it, the couple didn't have a lot of sex during the six months they dated before marriage. Joe accepted the situation because he thought that Chloe's Catholicism was the cause. He thought she was experiencing guilt over having sex outside of marriage. When they were on their honeymoon in Maui, Joe noticed that Chloe couldn't achieve orgasm during sex, but he generously believed that her enjoyment would improve over time and that eventually orgasms would be within reach. Unfortunately, the exact opposite happened. Instead of improving, the sexual side of their relationship worsened until it finally stopped completely.

Now, Chloe seldom allows him to touch her in a sexual way. She does love being in his arms, but she prefers physical contact that is platonic and romantic—without going any farther. Sex just doesn't interest her anymore. Joe on the other hand continues to want and need to engage in "having sex." Cuddling just doesn't do it for him. He fantasizes and dreams about sexual encounters, and abstinence is driving him crazy.

Clearly, their marriage is suffering. Chloe herself doesn't look happy. She used to be very joyful before marriage, but since the wedding, she is very often sad and tired.

As months have passed, they are both, in my estimation, sinking more and more deeply into depression. Both have been waking earlier than normal without being able to go back to sleep. When I see them, a defeated look appears to have etched itself into their young faces.

Depression often results from loss, and for Chloe and Joe the loss is in the mutual absence of sexual pleasure and intimacy. Depression also results from suppressed anger—in their case a mutual blaming for the loss of pleasure. Here I had to deal with both of the major drivers of depression.

But how can we find a way to cure this double whammy? Is a cure even possible? Can Chloe experience sexual orgasms? The Kinsey Institute estimates that only 8 percent of women have orgasm during penile/vaginal intercourse. This lack of sexual fulfillment leads many women to lose interest in sex, which often increases marital tension and is frequently a factor in infidelity and divorce. Marriage counselor and author Michele Weiner-Davis wrote:

"When one spouse is sexually dissatisfied and the other is oblivious, unconcerned or uncaring, and has no interest, sex isn't the only casualty; intimacy on every level becomes non-existent. Spouses stop touching affectionately, having meaningful talks, laughing at each other's jokes, or connecting emotionally. They become like two ships passing in the night. Infidelity and divorce become all too real threats."

If Chloe is unable to have orgasms, finding a way to help the couple will be difficult. I feel uneasy about this possibility but quickly put that worry out of my mind. Let's find out what is really happening.

I decide to try encouraging them to give their genitals a voice. As we've seen, I have used this technique with other patients, but with less taboo parts of the body. I know it will be a difficult concept for them to accept. I need to go slowly.

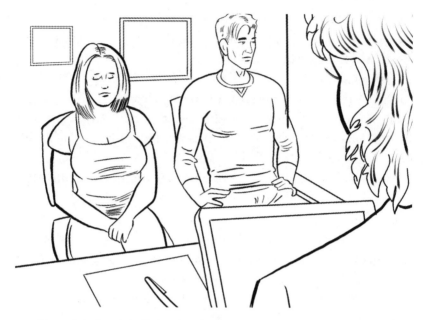

*"You might be sick all the time because you're not happy anymore.
Let's try giving your genitals a voice!"*

I start with Joe. "Joe, I'm going to ask you to do something that may seem weird and uncomfortable, but you'll understand why it's important in a moment."

Joe looks guarded, but he gives me a short nod.

I ask him, "If your penis had a voice—if it could actually talk—what would it say about its condition?"

Joe looks surprised, but takes a moment to collect his courage. Then he says in a halting voice, "I am Joe's Penis." He takes a deep breath, then presses on. "I am healthy, strong, and masculine. I need sex." Joe smiles sheepishly and pauses looking at me, seeking reassurance that what he is saying is okay.

I smile to show my approval. He is on the right track. "Great, Joe's Penis, continue talking! Tell us what you are experiencing on a day-to-day basis."

Joe, encouraged, continues: "Every morning, when Joe wakes up, I am really hard and big. Waking up next to Chloe is wonderful . . ." He glances at Chloe who is watching him and listening intently, "and I really want to be inside her, but she doesn't want me to touch her!" Glancing at Chloe again who is getting restless and blushing again, he continues, "At the beginning of our relationship, she did let me in, and it was great, although, it wasn't very often. She seemed to be enjoying herself, too. After the wedding, she seemed to have less fun, but I didn't care as long as I was happy. Now, she doesn't want me in anymore! She says she is too tired. She always says, 'Maybe tomorrow.' But then tomorrow comes, and she has a headache. She says it will be better by the weekend. The weekend comes and she has a stomach ache. . . . This is so frustrating to be sleeping every night next to my wife, wanting her so much, and not being able to have sex with her."

Joe's penis has said it all. Men's genitals are usually not too difficult to figure out. They want sex with their partners, which is understandable. They usually are very predictable with only one switch that is either on or off. Women's genitals, on the other hand, are much more complicated. They have several buttons that need to be pushed and knobs to be turned and tuned just right in order to get to orgasm. Is Chloe aware of that? Does she know her own body? Can she talk about that?

It is time to give Chloe's genitals their say. I suspect it will be much harder for them to speak, because women are socialized to be "nice girls" and mask their sexual needs. They have been taught that sexual needs are bad and unacceptable and can get them into trouble, especially if they are not married. Female sexual desires as a result can for some women remain bad and unacceptable throughout their lives—even when they are married. The needs and desires remain deep inside of their unconscious and are seldom allowed to come to consciousness and almost never allowed to have a voice of their own. But it is worth trying to give Chloe's genitals a voice. To start with, I know I need to be very subtle. I direct my attention to Joe. "I understand, Joe's Penis, that it is a very frustrating situation." Then I turn to Chloe. "Chloe, are you hearing what Joe's Penis is saying?"

Chloe, eyes downcast, nods.

"Now it's your turn, Chloe. Can you give your vagina a voice and answer Joe's penis?"

Chloe blushes. "I don't have any problem. Everything's fine."

Okay, I can see that she is closed up. I am not surprised. Most women are. How can I get her to open up?

"No, everything is not fine Chloe. Did you hear what Joe's Penis said? He isn't happy."

Chloe looks very uncomfortable. "I cannot talk about those things."

That's a very significant statement worth exploring. Who told Chloe she couldn't talk about sex?

"Why not? Why can't you talk about those things? Who told you that?"

"My mother told me having sex was bad, and my priest told me that talking about sex was not appropriate."

Ah here it is! Parental influence and church influence. In order to protect girls so that they don't have sex too early, parents teach them that sex is bad. The Catholic Church also teaches that sex before marriage is a sin. In itself, this teaching can sound reasonable to Catholics and others. The problem is that the association between *sex* and *bad* stays in some girls' minds so deeply engrained that they can't enjoy sex even after marriage. Sex remains associated with something bad forever. I have seen several similar cases in my office.

"Chloe, they were talking about sex outside marriage! Now you're married and that is very different! Sex with your husband is healthy and not sinful. It keeps him happy and fulfilled. And you also deserve to be happy and fulfilled!"

I can tell she is not receptive to what I am saying. It will be difficult to get her to talk about intercourse with Joe.

Maybe she will be willing to talk about masturbation? The clitoris is exquisitely sensitive with over 8,000 individual nerve endings packed into a very small area. A lot of women learn how to manipulate these sensitive areas and reach orgasm as they masturbate. They become used to touching themselves in a certain arousing way that men usually think they know about but often don't.

The other side of the picture is that some simply cannot have orgasms, but the numbers are small. Experts believe that fewer than five percent of women are anorgasmic, meaning they don't experience any orgasm through masturbation or with a partner, and they never will. I am hoping Chloe is not one of those women. The best way to find out is to ask her.

I am direct. "Have you ever masturbated?"

Chloe's face turns bright red and a little voice comes out of her. "I cannot talk about this."

The fact that she has blushed and declared her reluctance to talk about this probably means that she does masturbate. That is progress in our conversation. I have to be bolder now. I am probably going to shock her, but the topic is worth exploring.

"Okay, Chloe, I take that as a 'yes.' So, when you masturbate, you apparently do with your fingers exactly what your clitoris and vagina like. You know exactly the kind of touch that excites you. Have you ever told or shown your husband what the right touch is?"

Chloe opens her eyes wide and exclaims, "Oh no! I would never do that!"

Success! My bold approach is working. She just implicitly communicated that she knows exactly what is pleasurable for her, which probably means she can experience orgasms. I am relieved.

"Chloe, Joe has no idea how to caress you, kiss you, touch you. He can only take wild guesses that could easily be and probably are wrong. You are the only one who knows exactly how to touch yourself! You need to tell him and teach him!"

As I am finishing talking, Joe intervenes, confirming what I am saying: "Yes honey, this is true! I don't know how to please you. This is driving me crazy! I want to know what you'd like me to do!"

Chloe's face is now the brightest shade of red I have ever seen. Clearly she is very uncomfortable, but it's time to try again. "So Chloe, let me go back to my first question. If you could give your genitals a voice, what would they say?"

Chloe, with a little voice, asks: "Are you talking about my clitoris or my vagina?"

Ah, that's a surprise! Now I know she is going to open up! I am so glad. I just need to push her a little bit more and probably ask her to start with the voice of her clitoris, since she just mentioned it.

"Let your clitoris speak. Chloe's Clitoris: Welcome! How are you? What kind of touch do you need? If and when Joe is touching you, does it feel good or not?"

Chloe finally opens up and becomes willing to participate in this dialogue. She starts out by slowly choosing her words. "I am Chloe's Clitoris. I am very sensitive and delicate. I am used to soft pressure with some kind of vibrating oscillation that is very pleasurable. Joe often rubs me the wrong way or presses on me too much. It doesn't feel good. Instead of turning me on, it turns me off." As she finishes talking, Chloe turns pale and looks embarrassed.

Joe is listening intently, looking stunned, as if struck by lightning. It is obvious he had no idea that the way he was touching his wife was not pleasurable to her.

It is very frequently the case that women expect their man to know exactly where to touch them, when to touch them, and with what intensity. They expect their man to know how to push all their buttons the right way. This is usually an unrealistic expectation. Even though most men are tinkerers at heart, and know how to make things work, they have no clue how women's buttons function. Also since every woman is different, what they learned for one woman will not work for another. As a consequence, the only way for a couple to have satisfying sex is to talk and tell each other what works and what doesn't. But in real life, not so many women are willing to talk openly about this. I can see Chloe is already starting to close up.

I rush in. "Chloe's Clitoris, how do you want Joe to touch you? Do you want to spend the rest of your life without Joe touching you the way you like and deserve? He needs to know. Tell him!"

Chloe reflects in a whispering voice, "I love it when he places his warm tongue on me and presses on and off. He did that a few times on our honeymoon. There is a certain pressure I really like. If it's too much pressure, it hurts and turns me off. If it's too little pressure, I can't feel anything. It needs to be just right. Also the speed is important. It needs to be just right, not too fast, not too slow."

I glance at Joe. He is sitting quietly, mesmerized.

I continue addressing Chloe's Clitoris and ask what else it finds pleasurable.

I continue to emphasize that I am not directing my questions to Chloe but only to Chloe's Clitoris. This way, I continue bypassing taboos and defense mechanisms. I want to continue having uncensored access to raw primal needs that are still so vital in our human's life.

Chloe's Clitoris answers. "There is one thing that Joe did once that was wonderful. He put his lips together and applied some kind of suction on me. I am not sure exactly how he did that, but it was something I had never experienced before." Chloe's face is bright red from embarrassment or could it be from arousal?

Yes, I am thinking, this is something that men seldom know about. When suction is applied to the clitoris, its blood vessels fill up with more blood. This makes the clitoris more erect which creates intense pleasure. The same technique is also applied to penises when they have trouble getting erect. As a matter of fact, suction devices are sold for masculine erection dysfunctions. I am glad Joe is hearing all this.

Suddenly Chloe stops and shifts to her own voice. "Then I feel my vagina dilate, and I want him."

This is important, as she is now, without my encouragement, shifting the focus to her vagina. Joe has probably enough information now on clitoral stimulation to start researching the topic in preparation for the next time they are intimate.

I thank Chloe's Clitoris and direct my questions to Chloe's Vagina. I learn from it that Joe enters her too quickly, too deeply, giving her pain instead of pleasure.

"I need time to dilate and get ready for him. I want him to get inside me slowly, first staying at my entrance going back and forth in a very shallow way then going deeper and deeper in me as I dilate more and more." She stops talking, glancing at me and at Joe to see our reaction then focusing on the white floor again.

Now her vagina adds some detail: "Sometimes, he comes in at a certain angle, and if he does this with the right speed, it's wonderful. But very often he goes too fast in and out of me and with too much force. It is very painful."

Now it is time for me to create a dialogue between Chloe's vagina and Joe's penis. We are used to dialogues between our minds (for example when we speak with our partner in normal conversation our mind is talking to our partner's mind) but almost never do we bypass minds to have pure primal dialogues between vagina and penis. This kind of novel dialogue is usually very instructive because it gets to the heart of the matter.

With a big smile on my face I address both patients' sexual body parts. "Joe's Penis, give Chloe's Vagina your reaction to what she just said. And say what you would like from her."

Joe gives voice to his penis that says, "I am so sorry if I hurt you! That wasn't my intention. I just want to give you pleasure. I want to know all about what you like. It would be so much fun for me to explore things with you. Giving you pleasure gives me pleasure."

Chloe gives voice to her vagina that says, "I always thought that your own pleasure was more important than mine. I am so surprised you are willing to explore sex with me. I want slow

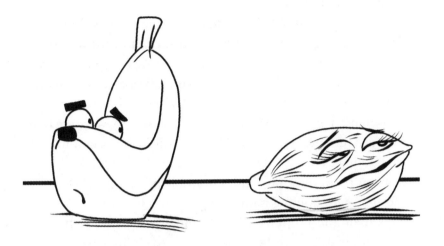

Banana: "I would love to play with you but I am sad and
frustrated because you don't want to play with me anymore!"
Oyster: "That's because you never touch me the way I like!"

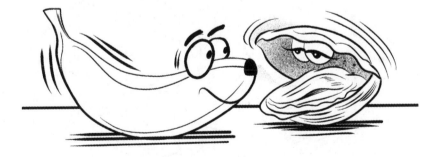

Banana: "Really? You never told me! Can you tell me what you like?
I'll do anything to make you happy!"
Oyster: "Oh! Thank you!"

movements. And maybe we can try different positions so that you can touch me in different ways."

The back and forth conversation between Joe's Penis and Chloe's Vagina goes on for a while with each other disclosing what they really enjoy and don't enjoy on a practical, primal level.

Here again, one person's body part talking directly to the other person's body part bypasses the brain and its taboos, embarrassment, negative self-criticism, and censoring. What we have left is pure fundamental needs that are still so important to us as human beings.

Both of them have big smiles on their faces as they leave my office. They are holding hands.

This dialogue between Chloe's and Joe's genitals changed their relationship and their life and saved their marriage. Joe learned about foreplay, about the kind of pressure and speed that would get Chloe excited.

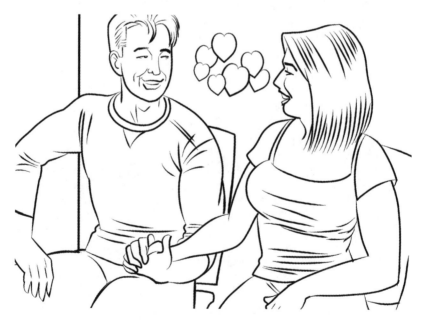

*Chloe: "I am so delighted you are open to discover what I like! Let's run home!"*

They began to have fun exploring sexual positions and found one that triggered maximum pleasure and orgasms for Chloe. She especially enjoys being on top of him. This way, she is the one in control of the speed and depth of penetration. She is also the one in charge of the angle of Joe's penis, making sure he is touching her most sensitive spot with just the right pressure each time they have sex. She's discovered that she is capable of powerful orgasms.

They have now been married for two years and are very happy.

Many women have similar experiences with their partners. They are unable or unwilling to tell their partners the details of what they really like. Their male partners have no idea of how complex a woman's body is or how to navigate it successfully.

But as we have seen, the direct conversations I have been able to encourage between partners' sexual organs can bring radical and often very enjoyable solutions. The same principle applies to same-sex couples.

Can my method be applied to other kinds of physical symptoms due to sexual dysfunction? I have found that it can. It can even work, as we will see in the remainder of the chapter, when one partner is unwilling or unable to have sex with the other partner under any circumstances.

One might think that by talking directly about sex we open a Pandora's Box of problems that might make distressful situations significantly worse. Perhaps this is why people are very shy about getting to the deep core of problems. What if no solution can be found? What if a partner opens up completely—body and mind, unconscious and conscious? What if all cards are placed on the table and the most horrible, impossible problems are uncovered? Will a downward spiral begin? Most people see such openness as taking a huge risk.

But my experience shows that it isn't. There is *always* a solution. I'd like to demonstrate this with the case of Ronald and Esther. Ronald arrives at my office for an evening appointment. He has complained of constant pain in his middle and lower back, and he is now looking for an alternative-medicine treatment. His medical history indicates that he has seen several physicians for his pain, has tried anti-pain and anti-inflammatory medications, but doesn't like the side effects, especially the stomach pain that the pills are causing. He is looking for a different kind of treatment.

He is a tall, good-looking, fifty-nine-year-old man. He is six feet two inches, one hundred ninety-two pounds, and comes into my office smiling and walking with his back long and straight.

I am immediately surprised by the discordance between his complaint of back pain and his smile and straight posture. As I welcome him to my office and offer him a seat, I pay attention to the way his body moves. My impression is that his back is flexible when he walks and sits down, so the pain probably isn't too intense.

Ron hands me his X-rays and MRI.

What I see doesn't surprise me: a little disc compression between "L5" and "S1," but not much. L5 is the last vertebra of the lumbar spine (just above the lower part of the spine), and S1 is the first vertebra of the sacral spine (lower part of the spine). The cartilaginous disc (made from cartilage and not from bone) in between them is usually the one that has to carry most of the patient's weight and has the most pressure on it. In many people after the age of fifty, even in people who have no pain at all, there is usually disc narrowing simply because of the force of gravity as we walk vertically. I have seen much worse disc compression with no pain. I ask myself the obvious question: "Why does Ron have so much back pain with so little visible damage?" I am guessing that other physicians whom Ron has seen have asked the same question without any obvious answer.

I am hoping that my unconventional approach to healing will provide Ron with some relief. I go ahead and begin to apply the technique that is often successful. I ask him to give his back a voice and to talk to me.

Since this approach is somewhat new to Ron, to put it mildly, I first ask him to describe and visualize his back in the first person. Was he (his back) born strong or weak? What is he (his back) made of? How big are his vertebrae? How strong are they? How is the cartilage that separates them? How are the muscles around his vertebrae? Are they relaxed? Are they tense? How are the nerves around his vertebrae?

Here is a summary of the answers given by Ron's back:

"I am Ron's Back. I was born sturdy and very healthy. I am made of big vertebrae with solid bone. My cartilages are robust. The muscles around my bones are powerful, maybe too powerful because they are tensed up and are squeezing the nerves around them."

Now that I have Ron completely focused on his back, I know that his consciousness is out of the way. Now that I have access to his *unconscious*, I can ask some key questions and address them to his back:

"Can you tell me, Back, why you are in pain? You are going to say that you don't know, but even if you don't, Back, what would you say? Don't think too much. Just say whatever comes to you, even if it doesn't seem to make sense."

This last sentence is the one that opens all doors. The fact that things don't need to make sense keeps away conscious thought, which often wants to make sense of everything. Having permission to say whatever comes up opens the door to the unconscious since sometimes the original reason for a body pain is not apparently linked to that pain.

After more exploring and more questions, Ron's back tells me, "My bones are strong but the muscles around my bones have spasms, painful spasms. They happen especially when coming back from work and spending evenings and weekends at home."

Ah, here we go, I think. He possibly has a stressful marital situation with his wife, Esther. I stop speaking to Ron's back and begin speaking to Ron directly. When I ask about the condition of his relationship with Esther I hear, "It is fine." All too often I have found that "fine" is really an acronym F. I. N.E. for Fucked-up, Insecure, Neurotic, and Emotional. Generally that means a sexless marriage. Sometimes no sex is the origin of a stressful marriage or sometimes a consequence. Either way, it still means no sex, which, as we know, is important for a healthy life.

I decide to ask more intimate questions. "Ron, do you argue a lot with your wife, and . . . how is the sex with her?"

Ron responds without hesitation. "No, we don't argue. As far as sex, what sex? There is no sex anymore, Doc. We've been married for thirty years!"

His answer does not surprise me. I have seen several cases of lower-back pain in men directly or indirectly related to sexless marriages. Men need sex to de-stress and enjoy life. Being denied sex makes them much more edgy with much more muscle tension, especially in their lower-back area. I am curious to know more.

"How long has it been?"

"About six years."

I continue to explore the issue. "What happened?"

"Six years ago, Esther was diagnosed with uterine cancer. Her uterus and ovaries were removed. We stopped having sex. I miss it a lot! But what can I do? I don't want to have an affair or see a prostitute. Marriage is for life, and I would never be unfaithful to her."

This is a twist I wasn't anticipating. When women go through pelvic surgery for cancer and, if necessary, radiation to burn any leftover cancer cells, it changes a lot of their pelvic anatomy. Surgery can destroy nerves, radiation burns delicate tissues, and intercourse becomes painful instead of pleasurable. Since there is no way to fix that, can a solution to Ron's problem be found?

I first need to make sure that the lack of sex is directly related to his muscle tension. "Could the lack of sex be the origin of your back problems?"

Ron is looking thoughtful now. "Possibly. I am very tense when around Esther. I love her very much. I am still attracted to her. I wish I could be sexual with her, but I know she doesn't want me to. It's a struggle for me every day."

This confirms my diagnosis. His "every day" struggle creates back pain. His body is suffering, and the anti-inflammatories he has been prescribed are just superficial and temporary help. A deeper fix is needed. When I ask Ron if he has talked to Esther about his problem, he explains that he hasn't because she is emotionally fragile. He doesn't want to cause her any upset.

I know now what I have to do. I must have them together in my office and expose Ron's problem to them as a couple. In that way, we will find a mutually acceptable solution.

Late that following afternoon, Ron and Esther are in my office. Esther is a very pretty woman in her fifties. She has blond hair, beautiful blue eyes, and a great smile. I have the immediate feeling it will be easy to talk to her. She is dressed very elegantly in an expensive-looking green suit, a white shirt, and high heels. Her look is in big contrast to Ron's wrinkled blue shirt, blue jeans, and tennis shoes.

I welcome them and begin with some polite exchanges of small talk. Then I dive right into the issue explaining that Ron's back muscle spasms are caused by a lack of sexual activity. I make clear that if we are to help get rid of his chronic back pain, we need to find a solution that is satisfactory to both of them.

Esther looks shocked and ill at ease, and I worry that this encounter may be too much for her to handle. I know that Ron has said that she is emotionally fragile, so I need to be gentle. I want to make sure she does not walk out!

I try to look confident and respectful at the same time. I tell her that I have seen many couples with similar situations of seemingly sexual incompatibility, and I explain my healing methods to her. I tell her that the best way to find a solution is to give Ron's penis and Esther's vagina a voice.

Esther appears very tense. I notice that she is looking at the door. I can guess that a part of her wants to run out of my office but another part of her, probably the one that cares for her husband, makes her stay.

It does seem risky to open this Pandora's Box of sexual issues because there is no obvious solution. But I am certain that being transparent and truthful will help us find a way. In my experience, problems usually arise when people want to avoid the truth, not when they dive into it.

Trusting me and my methods, Ron's Penis speaks: "I have the powerful urge to have sex. It's really difficult to control. It's built into me. I would like to have sexual intercourse with Esther but since she cannot have me anymore, I would like Esther's lips or hands on me. That will satisfy me and help me be happy. Otherwise, I am afraid I'll be drawn to other women."

I look at Esther. She is spellbound.

I thank Ron for letting us know what his penis has to say, and I tell Esther to give her vagina a voice in the same manner. She is extremely reluctant, but I explain to her how important openness and truth-telling is in this situation. After a few minutes of discussion, she is convinced and begins to speak. "I am Esther's Vagina. I have been really injured by the cancer surgery. I am small, tight, and not at all interested in being penetrated by Ron. I have tried to have his penis inside of me but the pain is too intense. My sexual time is over. I am sorry." Tears flood Esther's eyes.

Here is where the encounter can become risky if we continue past this point. It seems that we've arrived at a dead end, but my philosophy is that there are no dead ends as long as we are engaged in an honest journey towards the truth, whatever it may be. If so engaged, a solution will be found. But how do we look for it? Do I have the right healing secret in my bag of unconventional medicine?

I believe I do. The secret is to create a completely different point of view of the situation for my patients.

I ask Ron and Esther to stand up and accept the idea that the chairs they were sitting in as they gave a voice to their genitals still represent his penis and her vagina. Even though the chairs are now empty, I rearrange them so they are facing each other. Ron and Esther remain standing, and I ask them to turn and keep the chairs within their gaze. The effect is that they are now separated from their genitals—and their genitals' needs—and are able to view them in a neutral, detached way. The reason: We can be more objective when dealing with someone else's problems than when we are dealing with our own. By keeping the couple's genitals on the two chairs, separated from their owners, I effectively make Esther and Ron's sexual problems, for the moment at least, "someone else's problem." We now have five entities in the room: Ron's Penis (chair 1), Esther's Vagina (chair 2), Ron standing, Esther standing, and me, also standing next to them.

Once that setup is achieved, then and only then do I ask the question: "Ron and Esther, you have heard your genitals talking and expressing their needs and concerns." Pointing to Ron's chair, I say, "Ron's Penis needs sex." Pointing to Ester's chair I say, "Esther's Vagina doesn't want to be touched."

I continue. "Ron is getting tense and sick from receiving too little affection but doesn't want to be unfaithful to Esther because he loves her so much. What is the solution that you, Ron and Esther, can find as a couple that is truly acceptable to both of you? I am directing my question to you, not to the genitals."

The conversation between Ron and Esther that follows is very honest. They are exploring all the possible answers when I remind them that Ron's penis said he would be happy with just her hands or her lips on him.

Esther surprises everybody with her response. "Oh I would be very happy to use my lips or my hands. Until now, I really didn't want any physical contact because I didn't want intercourse, but if you understand and accept that I can't have intercourse, I would be very happy to give you oral sex."

Ron is very surprised and pleased, "Really, Darling? You would be willing to do that?"

Esther is smiling now. "Yes, Honey, of course! I had no idea that our lack of a sex life was causing your back spasms. I don't want you to be in pain because of me. I love you so much! You are such a wonderful husband."

That's it! They have found a fix to their problem. All that was needed was facing the blunt truth. It is crucial for our good health that we deal with what is *real* even if reality is different than what we think it should be. We can only truly cure illness when we address its true, deep causes. Otherwise we are dealing with fake and superficial problems that are solved with equally fake and superficial solutions that ultimately never work long term.

Ron and Esther leave my office that evening holding hands.

I see Ron the following week, and his lower-back pain is much alleviated.

This case shows that a symptom, like Ron's back pain, usually has a *reason* for being present. If the pain isn't explained by abnormal findings from X-Rays, CT scans, or MRIs, the pain has a purpose. My goal as a physician is to unveil that purpose. We all have different real needs in order to live happy, healthy lives. Some needs are easy to figure out and take care of; others are difficult and sometimes embarrassing. The differences are what make people interesting and appealing. And they certainly make my work as a physician challenging and fascinating.

As we saw in Jackson's case in chapter two, his back muscles had painful spasms because they were too immobile and needed stretching. He also needed to release anger by using a punching ball. Ron, on the other hand, didn't need stretching—he needed sex.

Individual vital needs are crucial to recognize and accept. If our vital needs are not met, medical symptoms will appear. If the symptoms don't somehow or someway get the body what the body needs, illness will develop. My job is to find and address the reason for symptoms as early as possible and find a fix that will prevent the illness from establishing itself.

## A Healing-Secret Exercise

Here is a practical exercise for you to explore your feelings about your "sex life."

PART ONE

Are you happy and fulfilled almost all of the time with your sexual partner?

If not, be aware of the symptoms you are having when you feel you want or need more sex or less sex or a different kind of sex.

Do you have muscle tension? Where is the tension?

Do you have aches and pains anywhere?

What are your feelings? Anger? Sadness? Frustration? Joy? How and where do they manifest physically in your body?

Make a mental note of all this.

PART TWO

Think about the person with whom you share your bed.

Then disconnect from your mind and give your genitals a voice. If they could talk, what would they say to your partner?

Complete the following sentences:

"Mr. Penis (or Ms. Vagina) really enjoys it when you . . ."

"Mr. Penis (or Ms. Vagina) would really enjoy things even more if you could . . ."

Let your partner know the results of this conversation.

Then, if willing, ask your partner to encourage her or his genitals to speak up with the same questions:

"Ms. Vagina really enjoys it when you . . ."

"Ms. Vagina would really enjoy things even more if you could . . ."

Next time you have intercourse with your partner, both of you can try to incorporate as much as possible his or her wishes as long as they are acceptable by both parties and not hurting anybody emotionally or physically.

As a result, your sex life will be more pleasurable, your orgasms will be stronger, your endorphins will increase, your stress will decrease, you'll have less aches and pains, and fewer infections thanks to a stronger immune system, less cardio vascular disease, better sleep, and your life will be more balanced and your longevity extended.

# 5

# Inner Group Therapy

I LOOK UPON THE body as a big family of organs. The different family members in this house are our heart, lungs, liver, spleen, kidneys, brain, legs, arms, back, and more. As with any family, all the members of the family need to live peacefully under the same roof, or in this case, the same body, and that isn't always easy because each member may have different needs, wants, and concerns.

Sometimes certain parts of our bodies have needs that are the opposite of, and thus incompatible with, other body parts, or as I am suggesting here, other family members. What happens then?

This results in conflict.

In the previous chapter, I showed how I was able to help my patients by having the body part of one partner interact directly with a corresponding part of the other partner. Using this technique we were able to uncover and address unfulfilled needs and wants that were causing or aggravating physical illnesses. I like to think of this technique as a sort of *couples* therapy.

In this chapter, I will move to a somewhat more complicated method I sometimes use that I liken to *group* therapy. You may be surprised to see who participates in the group.

In psychotherapy, patients are treated in groups of about six to twelve when they have interpersonal difficulties with multiple people—or people in general. Encouraging patients to interact with several others simultaneously can be very helpful for treating shyness, lack of trust, hostility, narcissism, and other problems that crop up in dealings with others.

I have found that group psychotherapy offers a very useful model for thinking about and treating *physical* illness in patients stemming from more complex problems than what I have presented so far in the book. Often patients come to see me with multiple physical ailments arising from several issues; for example, the inability to stop overeating results in obesity, and back problems are caused by the obesity. I see a situation like this one as "my stomach craves food, but my back suffers from my obesity, and my mind doesn't know how to resolve the problem!"

Such complex, intertwined problems present unique challenges as I bring my unconventional healing techniques to my patients.

Most people understand the difficulties that two-party interactions can cause (for instance, my body wants to have sex with that person in the next office, but my mind says I'd get fired for trying it). But breaking the mind and body down into multiple conflicting parts is not as easy.

So I convert an unfamiliar concept—multiple conflicting inner body parts—into a concept that is familiar to almost everyone: conflicts amongst a group of people. Who hasn't been part of a group with lots of hidden conflict and intrigue?

I call the techniques in this chapter "inner group therapy" because most people are familiar with the idea of groups comprised of individuals with different needs and goals.

There is an additional aspect of group therapy that is important here. I mentioned before that taking on the role of a different entity, such as our lower back, changes our perceptions, motivations, and judgments. Stanford Psychologist Phillip Zim-

bardo dramatically demonstrated this in his famous prison experiment, where students playing the role of prison guards
unconsciously took on so much of the personalities they'd been
asked to play that they actually became violent towards other students playing the role of prisoners. This development forced
Zimbardo to end the experiment before anyone was seriously
hurt.

Because we all have to show different sides of ourselves in different situations, and we are a highly social species, we are in a
sense, born actors.

I use our natural acting abilities throughout my work by getting patients to shift their definition of "I" from their minds to
their bodies, so that they can see things from their body's point
of view. When there are conflicts among multiple body parts, as
we'll see below, I also use this technique to get patients to assume
the role of an objective, highly rational personality I call the *Inner
Me-diator* who represents and expresses different points of view
and can ultimately resolve these conflicts.

I believe that we all have a conflict mediator inside us. We've
all been called upon at one time or another to settle conflicts
between family members or coworkers, or others around us.
When we are at our best, we do this in a rational, reasonable,
natural way. In my practice I bring out this mediator persona in
my patients so that the patients themselves can figure out how to
reach compromises between "warring" inner parts. I call this
healing secret *Inner Group Therapy.*

I used inner group therapy with a patient I'll call Florent.

Florent's relatively simple case involves giving a voice to his
mouth, kidneys, and heart. As we'll see, there is a conflict raging
inside him that only a wise inner part of him can solve: the Inner
Me-diator.

Then there is Robin's more complex case. She suffers from
puzzling, separate ailments. With the help of several colorful
pillows, she exposes her problems. She brings out her *Inner*

*Me-diator* to discover that all those seemingly separate diseases may be related, and that a simple solution can solve her medical problems.

In the next two cases, instead of giving a body part a voice, we will give a voice to a disease. In Lucia's case, her disease is cancer. Bringing the disease itself in the Inner Group Therapy will bring resolution to her inner conflicts. In our fourth case, we'll contrast her resolution with another completely different one made by Steve after giving his disease a voice.

Let's start with Florent's family conflict.

Florent is a happy-go-lucky person who enjoys life tremendously, but he has just awakened to the possibility that he may have been enjoying life a little too much. Florent has been eating very salty food his entire life, and now he has high blood pressure that is damaging his kidneys and his heart.

Before coming to me, he has a blood test that shows that his kidney function is worsening. His kidneys are having trouble eliminating all the sodium he is consuming.

As for his heart, the excess salt he has been ingesting is mixed with an equally large amount of fluid which is absorbed in his blood stream and arrives inside his heart with too much pressure stressing his heart more and more. His echocardiogram shows that his heart is bigger and his heart chambers more dilated than one year prior. Because of that dilation, his heart muscle is having more trouble sending oxygenated blood to all his organs.

But he is addicted to salty foods. His taste buds love salt. He needs help.

Florent's kidneys and his heart need a low-salt diet to survive, but his mouth craves highly salted food. These are opposite needs that create conflict.

How do we resolve the conflict?

First we need to expose the conflict by giving each party a voice. This means in Florent's case giving a voice to his mouth, his kidneys, and his heart. Florent is well aware of the basics of my methods and willingly begins to give voice to his mouth when I ask him to.

Florent, in a French accent giving voice to his already salivating mouth, "I love eating, Doc! Mmm . . . salty nuts, pretzels, ham, prosciutto, smoked salmon, parmesan cheese, onion soup! All so tasty! It's my biggest pleasure in life. It's true that I get thirsty afterward, but that's just a detail." His eyes are wide open, and he has a big smile on his face. Clearly he enjoys his food.

Hearing his mouth speaking, my first reaction is to laugh. He surely is epicurean like a lot of French people—and as I am. Pleasure from eating food is primal. Some people eat to live, and some others live to eat. The latter is clearly Florent's case.

But the problem is that every single food that he mentions has high-sodium content.

People don't realize that the body can get sick if its sodium intake is too high. The *2015-2020 Dietary Guidelines for Americans* recommend that Americans consume fewer than 2,300 milligrams (mg) of sodium per day as part of a healthy eating pattern.

I bet that Florent's salt intake is way higher than that. After eating loads of salt, he becomes thirsty as the body craves water to dilute the salt. Blood vessels swell up from a tsunami of salt and fluids. Blood pressure increases. Kidneys and heart become critically overloaded over time, and all this can be life threatening.

I need to make him see the big picture: the contrast between his happy mouth and his suffering kidneys and heart. It is time to give his kidneys a voice.

His face suddenly changes, becoming more serious. He seems worried as he says, "We, Florent's kidneys, feel a dull pain, which is probably due to our trying to eliminate all the salt Florent's mouth is eating. We've been to other doctors, and they say that too much salt is damaging us. They say we're at risk of kidney failure, which could lead to death." He looks at me with deeply sad eyes.

That is the reaction I am looking for. He is starting to get it. This is what I need to do to help him see the big picture the way

I see it, the way all doctors see it. While he gets it, I need to continue and ask him to switch and give his heart a voice.

Sadness stays in his tone as he gives his heart a voice. "I feel I'm beating too fast. Sometimes, I have palpitations and a sensation that I miss a beat. This scares me because I'm afraid I can't send enough blood to Florent's organs. The echocardiogram done last month shows that my cavities are getting bigger and cannot send blood as vigorously as they used to. I'm at risk of heart failure, which could lead to death."

His body posture changes. His shoulders slump and his face is drawn. I feel a palpable wave of sadness radiating from him, as if I have taken him to a precipice from which he can see his own death.

But this is Florent's reality! I have achieved what I wanted to achieve, and the family conflict is now exposed. One member of the family is doing something that is killing two other members—and that could get the whole family killed. Seems simple! But is it really?

We have exposed conflict but haven't resolved it. To resolve this kind of problem physicians usually give orders such as: You need a low-salt diet. Then they give the patient a sheet with a list of low-salt foods. Unfortunately, most patients don't follow such orders very well. This is just human nature. If I tell Florent he must switch to a low-salt diet, he probably won't do it. Or he might do it for a week or two before resuming his bad, perhaps fatal, eating habits. The solution needs to come from within him—from his "family."

Now, I must bring in another family member, The Me-diator, that neutral, wise part of us that can understand all family members and can make the most appropriate decision to satisfy all parties.

Sometimes patients confuse The Me-diator with their mind, because this is a thinking, reasoning, rational entity similar to what people commonly think of as their "mind."

But our minds aren't nearly as objective as we'd like to believe. Daniel Kahneman, the Nobel Prize-winning economist and psychologist, uncovered dozens of hidden biases that all of us unconsciously harbor. "Confirmation bias," for example, is our mind's tendency to interpret new data in a way that confirms already-held beliefs. If we like someone, we will not perceive their misbehavior as a problem but if we *dislike* someone, anything they do will be seen in a negative light.

In addition to hidden biases, minds have an agenda all of their own that compromises their objectivity. In the previous chapter on sexuality, I explained that many women's minds have been conditioned to believe that sex is nasty and even evil, making it hard for them to enjoy sexual activity. The mind wants to sustain the woman's view of herself as a "nice girl" versus a "bad girl." That mind cannot be a rational, reasonable conciliator in a conflict between, say, a vagina and the mind.

That's why it's important to create an entirely new persona, The Me-diator, whose only reason for being is to have no agenda whatsoever except conflict resolution.

I explain this in simpler terms to Florent and tell him that it is time to call upon his Inner Me-diator to find a solution acceptable to all parties.

I see that Florent is looking serious, really taking on the role of being his own mediator. After deep reflection, The Me-diator says:

"Well, I think the best solution is that from now on Florent eats a low-salt diet every day to keep his heart and kidneys from failing. But once a week he can have salty food so that his mouth can experience the salt pleasure from time to time." As he mentions that solution, his sadness seems to disappear. He looks pleased.

The Me-diator has come up with an interesting solution. It is a compromise that I wouldn't have thought about. Doctors generally don't think about making concessions to find a solution. They think about what's best for their patients' health.

They don't usually take into account quality of life issues and primal pleasures that are almost always the cause of treatment failures.

Nor do they think about the specifics of each organ.

The compromise that Florent's Me-diator has just found could only be created within him. Another patient faced with a similar problem would have found different concessions to make, ones that works best to satisfy all parties in *his* family.

Compromises that come from deep within are usually fully accepted and easier to implement whereas, as I said earlier—and studies back me up—orders from doctors are seldom fully followed.

Florent's decision made him very compliant with his new diet. As months went by, he became more and more accustomed to low-salt foods, and his once a week binge on salt became less and less pleasurable. As a result, he even stopped his scheduled bingeing in favor of sticking to the diet. As time went by, his blood pressure decreased. His kidney function improved. His heart stopped having irregular beats and became stronger. This whole process saved his life.

Solutions are not always so easily found.

Sometimes patients come to see me with a wide variety of symptoms that don't appear to have a connection with each other. The unconventional question I usually ask is: What if those different symptoms are somehow related? What if the answer is not to treat each symptom separately with different medications, but to see if somehow they are linked by an underlying thread that needs to be addressed if we are to find a long-lasting cure?

An example of such a case is my patient Robin.

Robin is one of my most knowledgeable patients as far as listening to her body and understanding it. She has been my patient for seven years, and I have treated her for many illnesses along the way. At times, it was just a cold or bronchitis, ailments that are easy to treat. Occasionally, she has more puzzling symptoms that are resistant to conventional treatments, like the occasional mysterious headache that began appearing a year ago.

In contrast to Florent, who understands and solves problems best by listening, Robin is a very *visual* person who grasps ideas and solves problems best by translating them into distinctive, concrete images. So to treat her, I use the same visual technique I used with Patricia, such as distinctly colored pillows to represent her body and her mind.

Like Robin, most of us are oriented toward the visual because forty percent of the most advanced part of our brain, the cerebral cortex, is involved with visual processing. So whenever I'm trying to get across a difficult or unfamiliar concept, my first approach is to translate the problem from abstract ideas into concrete visual symbols. In this way, the most powerful part of a patient's brain is helping separate out the various parts of the body we are trying to work with.

I have taught Robin to use different color pillows, to place them in a circle on the floor, and to sit on a different one each time she is working with a different part of her body to give it a voice.

My use of pillows to represent different parts of Robin's body is borrowed from the same Gestalt therapy method I previously talked about, called the "two chair" technique, in which patients are encouraged to "split" their identities into multiple parts in order to surface and resolve hidden conflicts between those parts.

Dr. Leslie Greenburg of York University has conducted numerous experiments showing that the two-chair technique is often more effective than other types of therapies at getting patients to discover and deal with emotional problems.

One reason for this success is that proxies for different parts of ourselves like pillows and chairs do not have the same automatic defense mechanisms such as denial that are in the conscious, thinking part of us that we normally think of as "our self."

Thus, the part of ourselves that sits on a pillow or a chair can connect directly to feelings and needs that our normal self has pushed deep below the surface.

We have seen this earlier in the Patricia's case, but there we were using only two pillows, one for her body and one for her mind.

The multi-pillow approach allows patients, by sitting in turn on each different pillow, to give each affected part of their body a full uncensored voice. I then ask them to take a step back and bring an extra pillow to the circle to represent their Me-diator, which then tries to find a solution to their problems.

Robin has gotten pretty good at that and rarely needs my help anymore, other than to write a prescription. For example, last winter when she had acute bronchitis after traveling to the East Coast to visit cousins, she used some pillows for a home session. After giving her lungs (that wanted to rest) and her mind (that wanted many social activities with minimal rest) a voice, she brought in her Me-diator who determined her traveling schedule was too packed and left her tired and prone to infections. Robin's mind decided she needed to take it easy and that she should take more time to relax in between social activities next time she traveled. She still came in my office for a prescription of antibiotics, and then took a few days off to rest.

One day, she calls me and asks for my help. I am curious to know what she needs me for. Since I pass her neighborhood on my way home, I decide to stop by.

Robin's house is small but has a gorgeous view overlooking a park and a little pond. A few seconds after I ring the bell, I hear a female voice "Please come in. I'll be there in a minute."

As I enter, I am pleasantly surprised by the smell of incense and the sound of soft, serene New Age music. The house is decorated with very refined taste. Two big brown leather couches are separated by an antique table. There are beautiful fresh pink, red, and yellow roses in vases. There are fine paintings on the wall, representing the ocean and peaceful sceneries of fishing villages in Asia. As I enter the living room my attention is drawn to several colorful pillows placed in a circle on the white carpet. I can tell Robin is having an Inner Group Therapy session.

"Are you doing your Group Therapy?" I ask with a loud voice and a smile on my face.

"Yes, I am," she says, shouting out of her bathroom "I can't understand what's going on with my body. I need your help!"

An attractive lady with shoulder length straight grey hair and brown eyes enters the room. She is sixty-five years old, but looks younger, about one hundred thirty five pounds, 5'5", and is wearing loose black pants and a striped black and white classy t-shirt.

She has a smile on her face, but I can see it is forced. She looks worried. "Why am I getting so many symptoms? They are starting to bother me when I teach my yoga classes. I want to get to the bottom of this! I tried organizing a group session between my head (she points at the white pillow on the floor), my fingers (she points at the yellow pillow), my skin (she points at the pink pillow) and my mind (she points at the colorful black, blue and white pillow), but I am getting nowhere. That's why I called you."

Robin is a great yoga teacher. I once took her class and, despite yoga not being "my thing," I really enjoyed her teachings. She has great positive energy when she is in the yoga studio but, somehow, in the class I attended, I could feel something was forced. There seemed to be sadness in her. I wondered if it was because of Kirk, her husband. She had been married to him for forty-five years and has had a good life with him. But he doesn't make her completely happy. Yes, he is a great provider financially, but he is not a great lover physically or emotionally. As a matter of fact, he is not a lover at all since he stopped touching her a long time ago. She told me in previous conversations that she was not really missing the sex, but she did miss the physical closeness and expressions of affection.

Ten years ago, she started complaining of red itchy plaques mostly behind her knees, inside her elbows, and on her belly for which she saw a dermatologist.

As years went on, the plaques got worse and were all over her legs. She was diagnosed with psoriasis.

Then, her fingers started to hurt, and the last joint of all ten fingers changed shape little by little, being more and more deformed. She saw a rheumatologist who prescribed anti-inflammatories.

Lately, she has been complaining of headaches, mostly in the evenings, starting around 5 p.m.

All blood tests and the brain MRI are normal. X-rays done on her fingers show degenerative arthritis. Her symptoms are manageable and she has learned to live with them, but why is her body acting up?

I am intrigued. I have worked with her in the past addressing sore throats, bronchitis, and fatigue, but I never addressed any of her arthritis, skin problems, or her recent headaches. They were looked after by her rheumatologist, dermatologist, and internal medicine physicians.

Could her headaches be related to her arthritis and psoriasis? That is an interesting question. The best way to find out is to do a group therapy session giving each sick organ a voice.

We begin a new session immediately. "What does your skin want to say?"

Sitting on the pink pillow, Robin gives voice to her Skin. "I am red and itching! I want to be scratched."

"Thank you, Skin! Now what do your fingers want to say?"

Robin now switches position, sitting on the yellow pillow and looking at her fingers. "We are hurting and looking ugly because of the deformity." She hesitates. "We want to scratch, but it is starting to be difficult because of the deformity." Her fingers are expressing the fact that being bent sideways because of the arthritis makes them more difficult and painful to flex when she is trying to scratch.

While listening to her, I begin to think about the situation with Kirk, her husband. I know she misses his affection. Maybe she needs to be touched. I wonder if instead of using the word "scratch," she uses the word "touch," some magical, unconscious door would unlock.

I say to her, "Can you start again? Sit on the pink pillow and replace the word scratch by the word touch and see what happens."

Robin gets off the yellow pillow and sits on the pink pillow again. "I am Robin's skin. I am red and itching because I want to be touched . . ." As she pronounces the word "touched" tears suddenly come to her eyes.

Yes! Robin's tears, arriving before she finishes her skin's thought, or even realizes that she is sad, is an example of the direct and immediate link between our limbic brain, that harbors unconscious emotions, and our bodies. In Robin's case, this strong link has just opened a door to her unconscious, and the resulting tears are a dead give-away that we have reached into a deep, very sensitive problem. Could this be the origin of all her symptoms? It is possible.

We needed a bridge between her symptoms and her emotions. Replacing the word "scratch" with "touch" did exactly that and bridged the gap between her unconscious and her consciousness.

She continues. "Oh my God!!!! It's so true!!! I want to be touched so much!!! Kirk doesn't touch me anymore! It's been almost ten years! Oh my God!" She looks at me with eyes brimming with tears.

Her deep emotion is very moving. I begin to think about my own life and how important it is to my emotional balance that my husband hugs me and holds me in his arms every day. His actions fill up my affection well and give me strength. I turn my thoughts again to Robin.

Now I want to try to determine if the lack of affection in her life can be the origin of her finger symptoms.

I ask her to switch to the yellow pillow and give me the voice of her fingers again. She thinks for a while and then exclaims, "We want to touch Kirk so much but he doesn't allow us to. We don't want sex; we just want tenderness, but he isn't interested in being physical anymore."

Now, indeed, we have the unconscious link between her skin problem and the arthritis in her fingers. But what about her headaches? Could they be linked to the same origin? We need to consult with her head. By "head" I mean not her mind or her thinking organ, but simply the part of the body that experiences the pain.

I ask, "Can you switch to the white pillow and see what your head has to say? Why is it hurting?"

Robin is starting to become aware of the whole picture. "I am Robin's head, and I want to be loved. I want Kirk to be romantic and to tell me that he loves me. He can't do it. I've tried many times to get him to show me some affection, but nothing works. If he can't or won't, maybe someone else will. But that means having an affair, and I don't want to do that."

What I am hearing doesn't seem to be coming from her body anymore, that is, not coming from the head, which is a body part and can have pain like any other body part.

Instead, what Robin just said seems to be coming from her conscious mind, from pure consciousness. And her mind wants to be in control over her head, her body, and her life. Since her mind wants to talk, we need to give it a voice too. I first have to make sure that it *is* her mind talking.

So I say, "Is this still your aching head talking, or is it your mind, the part of you that processes thoughts?"

Robin replies, "It's my mind."

"Okay then, sit on the pillow that represent your mind and let's hear what it has to say."

Robin looks at the colorful black, blue, and white pillow. "I don't like this pillow anymore," she says, and she replaces it with a dark brown pillow. She sits on the new pillow and starts, "I am Robin's mind, and now I understand why you guys, Skin, Fingers, and Head, (she looks at each of the other pillows in turn) are hurting. But I can't leave Kirk! We've been married for forty-five years. He is an excellent provider. I love my home, and he pays for it! I could not afford it on my own. I love the fact that I can be a yoga teacher without having to worry about making money. I am financially safe with him."

At last! Now we have the whole picture. Everything makes sense. We have found a common origin for all her symptoms. Here is a possible explanation for all her symptoms: Lack of affection triggers stress which increases secretion of adrenaline, which constricts blood vessels, and cortisol, which weakens the immune system and inhibits the repair mechanisms of cells. If the stress continues, skin and joint damage that frequently happens in all of us will not be repaired, and damage is likely to become chronic.

We are making progress. We found a common origin for all of her ailments. We now need a fix.

We've given a voice to her skin, her fingers, her head (body part) and her mind. Now it is time to bring out her Inner Me-di-ator, the part of her that is neutral, understands all parties, and can help make the best rational decision.

Robin gets up, grabs a new pillow. This time, she seems to like the colorful black, blue, and white pillow. She makes a place for it in the pillow circle. Then she sits on it, remaining silent.

I remain silent too.

These are the golden minutes when I have to step away. I must allow her to take a step back, grasp the deep origin of her medical problems, and find a solution that can work for her, not for anybody else. It must be for her only. My role is to guide her, but the real work can only be done by her.

Everybody is different and two people faced with the same problem will find different solutions.

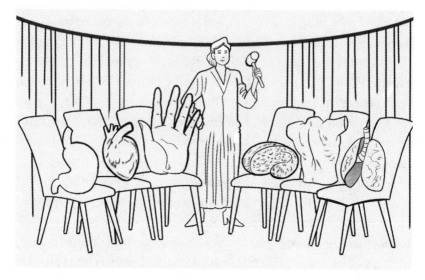

*Me-diator (with gavel): "Let's hear from each of you, organs! Stomach goes first—then Heart, Hand, Brain, Back and Lungs! Let's start!"*

Understanding people and treating their problems takes time. I need time to examine and work through the issues, and my patients need time to understand where we are going and to participate in the process. That's why a fifteen minute office visit doesn't make sense to me. Yet, that's the average time doctors and patients are allowed in the typical family practice. I usually like to keep patients for one hour. The benefits of a long office visit (or a home visit as in Robin's case) are incalculable.

After what seems at least five minutes, but in reality was probably only one minute, The Me-diator in Robin shakes her head before saying, "I understand the situation now!"

Looking at the pink pillow her Me-diator says, "Skin, you want to be touched, caressed and loved. That is why you are itching." Then switching her attention to the yellow pillow, "Fingers, you want to touch and be touched and love and be loved by a man, preferably Kirk! You have been dying for physical affection for so many years but have only met rejection. That is why you are deformed!" Switching her attention to the white pillow, "Head, you want to hear love words and to be with a romantic man but you can't. That is why you are hurting. Mind, you want to stay with Kirk because he is a good provider, allows you to live in a beautiful house, and be safe financially."

After a pause, her Me-diator continues, "That is a big dilemma. It was one against one a few years ago (Skin against Mind), then two against one (Skin and Fingers against Mind), and now three against one (Skin, Fingers, and Head against Mind). That means that you, Body, really need touch and love, but leaving Kirk is too risky. We don't even want to consider that." She pauses again and thinks deeply.

I choose to remain silent. I can do no more. She now needs to come up with a solution on her own.

After what seems a long time, her Me-diator announces, "I think getting a massage twice a month would be acceptable."

I am a bit surprised at this possible solution. I'm not sure what I was expecting, but at least now we have something to work with.

Now the task is to find out if the massage idea is acceptable to all parties, because it is important to respect all members of the body's family, just as we would in any kind of family therapy.

Robin seats herself on each pillow in turn for a few seconds to answer the critical question that must be addressed to each of her body parts: "Is the solution acceptable to you?"

I begin the questioning. "Let's ask Skin, Fingers, and Head if a massage twice a month would be a satisfactory solution."

Robin sits on Skin's pillow. "Yes, I guess it could be a temporary solution."

Robin moves to Finger's pillow. "Yes, this could work short term."

Robin sits on Head's pillow. "Yes, I guess, but I can't see your masseur murmuring love words." Robin bursts out laughing. "Oh well, better to laugh about it than cry!"

I too laugh. It's a good thing to mix a little humor in with the medicine, although it is clear that Robin's head is not going to be satisfied with the masseur solution for very long. I even doubt it will work on a short-term basis. But it is a good start. I am proud of Robin. She is a good student.

Now that she knows what is happening in her body, she won't be helpless anymore. She has some control of her situation. But I still worry about her. I have seen people getting sicker and sicker, piling up symptom on top of symptom because they didn't get along with their partner and chose to stay in an unhealthy relationship.

As I leave her, I think to myself, "It is amazing how much power our body can have! When its needs aren't met, it finds a way to let us know!"

There is even an emerging medical field called psychodermatology that is researching the relationship between mental problems and skin problems. It offers hints about why Robin's skin developed severe lesions in response to the stress of isolation and lack of intimacy with her husband.

In psychiatry, problems such as Robin's, in which emotional distress is vented and expressed through the body, are viewed as symbolic ways that patients communicate their angst to themselves and to the world.

According to the theory, Robin was communicating specific unmet needs for touch and intimacy. She craved touch in the very places her skin became inflamed: her legs, stomach, and arms.

Her skin was essentially screaming "Hey, touch me tenderly here, now!!!"

Although Freud and other early psychoanalytic thinkers based their beliefs about symptoms like Robin's on intuition and observation, recent research suggests that hard science may back up these intuitions.

For example, we now know that in addition to our skin communicating with our brain through sensory fibers (involving touch, temperature, or pain), our brains also communicate *to* our skin. Our autonomic nervous system (the part of our nervous system that is under unconscious control) can command targeted patches of our skin to sweat, small hairs to stand up (goosebumps), or blood vessels to constrict or dilate. Nerve endings in our skin also secrete substances that affect immune response and inflammation.

Sweat has also been shown to inhibit growth of some types of bacteria while causing other types to proliferate. Changes in bacteria cultures can also trigger local immune responses that promote skin inflammation.

These recent neuroscience findings demonstrate that all of the many unconscious neural and biological connections between Robin's brain and Robin's skin could have combined to produce the chronic inflammation.

What is Robin's situation now, a few years after the memorable session I've described?

She is still with Kirk and is still dealing with the same symptoms, but thanks to regular massages done by a good looking male masseur, and acupuncture done by a male acupuncturist, they are less intense and not interfering anymore with her teaching yoga.

Robin's case is a great example of how giving different body parts a voice can solve problems the way no physician, even the most competent specialist, can.

Usually in such cases, physicians provide what I call Band-Aid medications that may provide temporary relief but don't address the deep origin of symptoms. How could they? Doctors only have fifteen minutes to say hello, listen to your complaint, examine you, prescribe tests and medications, answer your questions, and write their note on their computer. They often have four patients per hour which means over thirty patients a day. It is difficult for them to take time to see the big picture. It is certainly impossible on a practical level for them to organize inner group therapy sessions, even if they were aware that such healing methods existed.

With Robin, I used group roundtable discussions involving body parts only.

I have found that sometimes it can be helpful to include the patient's disease itself in the group roundtable discussion. Giving the disease a voice and thus a place in the pillow circle is a different technique I have found very effective.

I use this different method with my patient, Lucia, who has cancer. She is undergoing heavy chemotherapy to treat her breast cancer and is suffering from chemo-induced intense nausea.

Lucia is forty-two years old, and despite the fact that she has lost all her hair and is looking very tired, I can see she is a beautiful lady. But she is so sick and tired of her toxic chemo that she is ready to give up, stop all treatments, and enjoy life again, even for a short time, even at the cost of succumbing to the cancer and dying.

As our session begins, Lucia's stomach is the first part of her body eager to have a voice. Lucia sits on the green pillow. The voice is angry. "I'm Lucia's stomach. I used to be healthy, strong, and I enjoyed spicy food. Now I'm nauseous all the time. Foods I used to love taste bad to me now. Foods that I used to digest well, cannot be digested anymore. I have painful spasms day and night. Life isn't worth living anymore. I hate this chemo that's making me sick. I'm ready to stop it and never take it ever again."

There is so much anger and so much energy behind her words that I have her shout "Stop Chemo! Stop Chemo! Stop Chemo!" to get the destructive energy out of her body.

She shouts with so much strength that the air is electric. I am feeling her pain. Her plight touches me very deeply. Chemotherapy for cancer really is horrible. In some cases, we bring patients to the border of their own death to kill cancer cells with no certainty that the treatment will cure them. The chemotherapy for cancer currently in use is archaic. In the future, we'll probably have much better treatments with far fewer side effects. But we are not there yet. Lucia's chemotherapy is the only possible treatment we know of today.

As often happens with cancer patients, Lucia's outpouring of suffering brings up conflicting emotions in me. On the one hand, I strongly feel Lucia's emotional pain and don't want to force her to continue the treatment and the suffering, especially since the chemo might not ultimately save her life. Sometimes quality of life is more important than quantity of life.

But a stronger part of me needs Lucia to beat her cancer, and I fervently hope I can help her do it.

Perhaps there is no more gut-wrenching decision a doctor has to make than whether or not to suggest to a patient like Lucia that "Enough is enough. You should start to get your affairs in order."

But I am not there yet, and neither is Lucia. So my goal now is to energize her and steel her for the struggle that lies ahead.

When most of her energy from her outburst has been expended, I instruct Lucia to get up, choose another pillow, and give a voice to her breasts.

She chooses a pink pillow and sits on it. Her face changes. Anger seems to leave her. The voice is now gentle. "I am Lucia's breasts. We are soft, beautiful and full of love, but are being invaded by this monster cancer. We are under attack and we are scared. We need help! We need somebody to protect us and kill the cancer." The voice is breaking as she becomes emotional. Tears are filling up her eyes. She pauses.

I give her time to process everything that is happening. Since silence is settling in, I say, "Is there anything else you, Breasts, want to say?"

She reflects then, "Not really, except . . . we hope we'll be healthy again soon." She looks at me with sadness in her eyes.

Her sadness touches me deeply. I have tears in my eyes too. I share her pain, and I share her hope. But this is not a time to get too emotional because I need to move Lucia's point of view away from herself and her suffering and onto her cancer.

So, adopting a somewhat brisk, professional tone to mask my emotion, I say, "Let's complete the circle and pick another pillow for cancer."

She reluctantly picks up a black pillow.

This is another one of my secrets. When our body is fighting against an enemy, it is very revealing to experience sitting in the enemy's shoes and experiencing the enemy's point of view. The technique may expose its strengths and weaknesses.

As in warfare, the way to victory is to know your opponent well, even to the point of befriending the enemy to learn its strong points and weak points.

Then, the next step is to attack those weak points. That usually ensures victory.

It's time to get to know Lucia's cancer.

Lucia reluctantly sits on the black pillow. "I am Cancer. I am strong and dark. I want to kill Lucia. I am invading Lucia's breasts and then will take her whole body."

Now I must look for the enemy's weaknesses. Lucia's cancer is inside her body so her unconscious probably has insights about the interaction between chemo and cancer.

I ask, "Cancer, what is your reaction to the chemo? Is it affecting you at all?"

Lucia is sitting very still. Then her cancer speaks, "Yes, it is hurting me. I hate chemo. It's destroying me. I can feel my cells disintegrating one by one. I can't invade Lucia's body anymore. It is paralyzing me."

Lucia suddenly realizes the power of the experience I have put her into. "Oh my God, the chemo is really working! The cancer is being knocked down. It's amazing!"

She seems mesmerized, and she stares at me.

I smile at Lucia, pleased with our results. They prove again that the body knows more than we think it does. But it is time to continue the exercise.

"Let's bring your Inner Me-diator in! Choose another pillow and bring it in so it closes the circle."

Lucia gets up and places a teal blue pillow in the circle. We now have four pillows in our inner group therapy: a green pillow for Stomach, a pink one for Breasts, a black one for Cancer and a teal blue one for Me-diator.

I ask her to sit on the teal blue pillow and become the Me-diator. As she sits, her voice becomes deeper, and she speaks more slowly. "I am Lucia's Me-diator."

I address the Me-diator. "You've heard Lucia's stomach. It is sick and tired of being nauseated by chemo. Then you heard Lucia's breasts say that they are invaded by the cancer. Then you heard Cancer itself, saying that it wants to kill Lucia but is being prevented from doing so by chemotherapy. It said that it is being destroyed by the chemo. What is your take on the situation, Me-diator?"

Lucia's voice is deeper and louder now. She is addressing the black pillow. "I understand the situation. I see that chemo is really working and destroying, you, Cancer." Then to the green pillow, "I know it's making you sick, Stomach." Now she points to the pink pillow. "But it is saving you, Breasts."

She pauses.

I remain silent and watchful. Each time I place one of my patients into a similar session, I never know what she will decide to do. Watching her move to a decision is a riveting, emotional experience.

Lucia continues in the voice of Me-diator. "Doctors don't know any better way yet, so chemo is the only treatment right now. It's slaughtering cancer cells and saving Lucia's life. It's worth having the side effects for a few more months. I vote for continuing chemo. Brace yourself, Stomach, it will be a wild ride. But in a few months, everything will be over and Lucia will be back to life, healthy and cured."

Lucia stops talking and takes a few deep breaths. Her Me-dia-tor has grasped the problem and presented a good solution.

When she gets up from the Me-diator pillow, Lucia is ener-gized with hope and resolve and willingness to tough it out.

Had I told her bluntly at the beginning of the office visit that she needed to continue chemo (which is what most doctors would have done) her body would have rebelled. She had to ex-perience deeply the whole scenario and come to the conclusion to continue chemo by herself.

This session led her to stick with the chemo. She was able to tough out the side effects and bravely go through surgery and radiation therapy. Now she is cured and enjoying life.

In Lucia's case, chemo was effective, but sometimes it is not successful. We now have genetic testing that allows us to see whether or not a particular chemo is going to have a potent effect on the target cancer cells. The testing can save patients from a lot of painful and ineffective trial and error, as cancers are often re-sistant to different forms of chemotherapy. But some doctors and institutions are still not using this genetic testing. People need to be aware that genetic testing exists and, if it isn't offered to them, they need to request it.

But what if chemo works for a short time and then stops work-ing? Well, our body will be the first to know. It will be aware of the failure much earlier than our physician. That's why it's important to know our body well and to listen to and understand the multi-ple clues it gives out about its health.

My late husband, Steve, is another example of a patient fight-ing against cancer who, when he listened to his body, found in-sights that were very different from Lucia's.

He was treated with chemo for his brain cancer. The drug worked well for one year, but then his body became aware that the drug stopped working. His physicians wanted to continue the treatment, but his body knew that was a mistake. His body knew sooner that his doctors, sooner than any MRI.

His clue: His right hand was starting to weaken. It was clear to him that his left brain was being attacked by cancer cells as it had been before the chemotherapy began (the left brain controls the right side of the body). His body showed no doubt about the treatment's loss of effectiveness because his symptoms were getting worse.

I have learned to listen to my patients' bodies. It is another one of my secrets, although I wish it weren't such a big secret unknown to the medical profession. If an X-ray or an MRI result is questionable, by asking the patient what the symptoms are, by actively listening to what the body is saying, and understanding what the symptoms mean, we can catch the problem early. Then we know that we must alter the patient's treatment.

In Steve's case, since his right hand was starting to weaken, he was sure (and so was I) his cancer was thriving again. This led us to arrange an earlier appointment with his cancer doctor. A brain MRI was done that showed a debatable progression of the cancer. The result of the test was enough to arrange an immediate change in the type of chemo, which extended Steve's life.

Being aware of what our body has to say can help us attack medical problems as soon as they arise. The sooner the problems are addressed, the easier they are to solve. That's how it worked for Carter, a victim of colon cancer.

Carter was sixty-six years old when he became aware of passing softer than usual stools with more abdominal gas. Carter's doctor scheduled a colonoscopy that revealed a colon polyp starting to transform into colon cancer. The polyp was removed right away, and Carter was placed out of danger. He is now eighty-two years old, healthy, and looking as young as ever. If he hadn't been aware of this change in his bowel movement, cancer would have been discovered much later, perhaps after it had metastasized, and it could have killed him.

Being in tune with his body saved Carter's life.

## A Healing-Secret Exercise

*Here's a practical exercise in group therapy:*

Let's do a group therapy session with your lungs, stomach, and lower back. The goal here is to increase body awareness. Have four pillows with different colors readily available.

Choose a pillow of your choice to represent your lungs and sit on it. Close your eyes and take a few deep breaths.

Feel how much your lungs expand when you inhale; feel how much air comes out when you exhale. Feel how warm or cold the air is.

Give your lungs a voice, describing what they are feeling here and now. For example, the lungs might say, "We feel how we are filling up with air and how pleasurable it is for us to expand fully."

Then describe what it feels like to exhale. Stay in the moment and describe it. Let your lungs talk as much as they want. Don't censor anything as long as you stay in the present moment. If your mind starts drifting off to other topics, bring it back to your lungs.

When you are finished, get up from your lung pillow and choose another pillow of your choice to represent your stomach. Put it not too far apart from the first one so that you can start a small circle. Sit on the stomach pillow.

Close your eyes and describe what your stomach is feeling. For example, you stomach might say, "I am so full and distended. There is too much food inside of me." Or it might say, "I feel empty. I need food." Or express whatever comes to mind as long as it describes your stomach's present moment.

When your stomach doesn't have anything more to say, get up and choose another pillow of your choice to represent your lower back. Place it down to continue the circle and sit on it.

Close your eyes and describe what your lower back is feeling. For example, it might be, "I feel stiff," or "I feel very flexible and painless," or whatever comes to mind. Stay in the here and now and describe the present moment.

When your back is done talking, get up and pick up the fourth pillow. Place it down to complete the circle and sit on it. This is your Inner Me-diator pillow.

Keep your eyes open, and with your Me-diator's eyes, talk to each pillow commenting on what it said. Talk to your lung pillow, your stomach pillow, and your lower back pillow. For example, you might say, "Lungs, you are breathing well, and it was a pleasure to listen to what you said. Stomach, you seem too full. You need to eat less in the future. Lower back, you seem in good shape," or whatever comes to mind.

You can do this exercise with any body part that you want.

This exercise will allow you to be more aware of what is going on in the different parts of your body here and now.

It is also a great meditation tool that allows you to slow down and de-stress.

# 6

# Speaking Through Dreams

So far I have described different techniques that allow patients to reveal feelings they may not even know that they have. These techniques are critically important because hidden emotions don't really go away. As we have seen, they very often surface as physical illness.

All of my secret healing techniques have one thing in common: They work their way around psychic defense mechanisms that stand between patients and awareness of the true cause of their suffering.

We have seen throughout the book that as I probe for deep truths, sometimes I have patients role play a body part that speaks out directly to me. Other times I set up internal dialogues between the body and the mind. And still other times I guide patients into internal group therapy among multiple body parts.

It's paradoxical, in a way, that I coach patients to step outside of themselves in order to get them in touch with what's going on inside of them!

A close friend of mine put it this way: "I don't know who discovered water, but it wasn't a fish!" In other words, we are all like fish who have never known anything other than the "water" of our emotional lives.

Just as fish have never experienced land or air, we humans almost never get to experience what it's like to live a life where we do not deny or repress emotionally uncomfortable or forbidden feelings. The reason we don't is that evolution has hardwired psychic defense mechanisms, such as denial and repression, deeply into our brains to help us avoid emotional distractions that could be fatal in the primitive, savage world our ancestors once lived in. So getting around hard-wired defensive circuits in the brain is not easy.

Our defense mechanisms are primal and strong, so sometimes I rely on techniques that appear to patients (and their unconscious minds) to be much less threatening than giving voice to a body part expressing strong emotion. I call these techniques "symbolic role-playing" to distinguish them from the role-playing methods I've described so far.

As we will see in this and in the two chapters that follow, symbols such as dreams, nature, and art can be incredibly powerful vehicles to take patients into the heart of their emotion and to ultimately heal their bodies. In this chapter I focus exclusively on symbolic role-playing in dreams.

I did not discover the concept that our unconscious speaks to us through symbols in dreams. It is not a new idea. Freud, Jung, and other Psychoanalytic theorists explored these areas long before me.

Gestalt therapists, whom I've discussed earlier in the book, also work with dreams, but differently from Freudian psychiatrists. Freud and others used dreams to explore repressed emotions about past traumas. Gestalt therapists focus on here-and-now experiences and emotions, believing that thoughts and feelings in the moment are most accessible and useful.

I'm going to describe briefly Gestalt dream therapy because it is the inspiration for the dream techniques that I use with patients when we are having a hard time getting to the source of their physical illnesses.

In Gestalt dream therapy, therapists ask patients to describe a recent dream, first from their own point of view, then from the point of view of what Gestalt therapists often call actors, sets, and props in the dream. For example, a patient who dreamed of meeting her father at a train station just as a train was pulling in, would be coached to, in effect, rewind the dream and replay it from the point of view of the father (an actor), the train station (a set), and the train (a prop). While role-playing each different element of the dream, the patient uses the first-person "I" and describes, at each step, how she is feeling in the moment as that particular part in the dream.

Gestalt therapists take this approach because they believe that when we are unhappy, we create the actors, sets, and props that appear in our dreams out of parts of our own personalities that are emotionally troubled, in conflict, or have other "unfinished business."

Thus when we take on a role and become a different part of our dream, and describe that part's emotions in the first person, we directly connect to repressed emotions. For instance, the patient might discover that when becoming her father in the dream, the father voices the feeling of regret for always criticizing the child's lack of achievement in school. That reveals that the patient carries within her a merciless critic who can never be pleased.

Exposing patients to such repressed emotions is how Gestalt therapists bring painful feelings out into the open so that they can be discussed and dealt with. In many cases, this promotes emotional healing.

But as a primary care physician, my ultimate goal is to heal the body, not only the psyche. So I have extended Gestalt dream work to encompass the physical body as well as the psyche.

I do this by asking one additional question that Gestalt psychotherapists do not traditionally ask: "Is there a direct link between the emotional pain revealed through a dream and the specific physical illness that a patient has when coming to me for help?"

When people come to see me with a chronic, difficult-to-treat symptom that coincides with a recent recurrent dream, I like to take them on a journey through their dream to explore a possible unconscious common origin. Maybe a repressed emotion expressed through their dream is also the one causing their symptom. Getting the repressed feeling out in the open and addressing it might be the missing key for a cure. I'll show you it works in two intriguing cases where, at first sight, a dream had nothing to do with the symptom.

First, we'll focus on Allison's simple case of knee pain. Then we'll explore a more complex case of a woman named Claudia who is complaining of chronic headaches. We'll take you on a riveting journey to find a possible emotional origin of her headaches through her recurrent dreams. I'll also disclose yet another of my secrets: *How revealing a repressed negative emotion can turn it into a positive healing emotion.* Then we will turn to a practical exercise that can easily be done at home.

Let's start with Allison.

She is twenty-one years old when she comes to see me complaining of right knee pain. The pain had started four weeks prior to her visit. An X-ray and a knee MRI are all normal, yet, she is having trouble walking. The most plausible explanation, given her young age, is that she probably has fallen or injured her knee while jogging. (Her chart says she has been jogging frequently.) But when I ask her, she says she didn't fall and had stopped jogging several months before the knee pain started.

I take in her general condition as she explains this to me, and I am already looking for other common causes of knee pain. She is short and has a little fat on her hips, but I wouldn't say she is overweight. So weight isn't the cause of her knee pain. Sometimes, people put on too much weight creating pressure on their hip, knee, and ankle joints. The pressure can compress the knee cartilage and create pain.

Allison has short curly red hair, her skin tone is fair, and her face has cute dimples that make her look very attractive. Her green eyes are hidden by round glasses with red frames. She is wearing a red shirt and a black short skirt that exposes her knees. I am already looking at her right knee. It doesn't look bigger than the left one. I am checking for redness (which would indicate inflammation) or black and blue color (which would indicate history of fall or other kind of direct trauma) or deformation (from birth, some people have legs that are arched out as if they are riding a horse or arched in with knees touching each other when they stand straight—either of which could give knee pain) but I see none of those.

My eyes continue wandering down her body as she speaks, looking at her calves and feet to check for any swelling. She is wearing flip flops that are exposing very normal-looking feet. I wonder if she wears high-heeled shoes (another possible cause of knee pain in a young female) on a regular basis. High heels change the point of body pressure impact at the knee level. I ask her about this, but she denies frequently wearing high heels.

She says she doesn't want to take any pain pills but wants acupuncture, a healing technique I offer my patients.

Now I am ready to examine her.

As I ask her to step up on my examination table. I notice she does it very easily with no pain. I first touch her knee with the back of my hand. The back of the hand is cooler and much more sensitive to heat than the palm of the hand. When checking a child for fever, we apply the back of our fingers to the forehead of the child. Remember that the palm of the hand is warmer. With Allison, I want to determine if there is any difference of temperature between the two knees. I find none, which means that there is no obvious inflammation.

I then ask her to relax and let me move her knee so that I can examine her range of motion. Trying to flex and extend her knee with my hands, I notice that it is unusually difficult to do so. She seems tense. I ask her to relax again, but she has a lot of trouble doing so. This is perplexing, and I make a mental note of this.

I complete my examination, and not finding any physical problems, I begin to wonder if there is an emotional component to her knee pain.

I set the thought aside for the moment and take some sterile acupuncture needles and rubbing alcohol out of my cupboard.

I place ten needles on her body, and since they need to stay in for twenty minutes, I set my timer and then decide to use that time to ask her a few questions.

"I am wondering why your knee hurts! Are you sure you didn't bang it or twist it some time ago?"

"I don't know, Doc," she replies, "I don't understand why my knee could possibly hurt... unless . . ." She pauses, and as a thought seems to come to mind, she laughs.

"Unless what?" I ask.

Allison is still laughing. "Unless I hurt it in my dream. But that was just a dream."

Ah ha! I feel a little thrill of excitement, at her mention of a dream. Sometimes a dream can help zero in on the cause of a symptom.

Casually, I ask, "Tell me about your dream. Did you have it last night?"

"Yes, and I frequently have this exact same dream. It's rather scary."

A recurring dream! She's got my full attention. I love recurrent dreams, the open door to the unconscious. We do have some time left in the appointment to do a little Gestalt interpretation.

I ask her to tell me about the dream in the first person and present tense (in other words, from her own point of view), which she gladly does. "I am driving a new car on an unfamiliar road when suddenly the road slopes steeply downward. I try to press on the brakes, but they don't respond. The road is now at a seventy degree angle, extremely steep. I try frantically to press on the brakes; then I try the emergency brakes, but nothing is responding. There is a big abyss below. I am going to go over it.

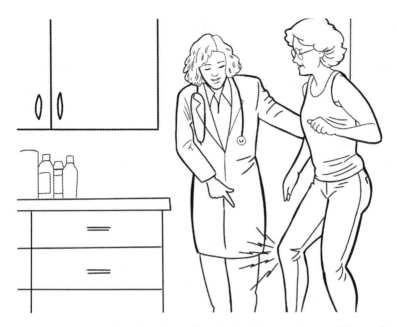

*Allison: "My knee has been hurting for four weeks, and I haven't been sleeping well because of a recurring dream!"*
*Doctor Chris: "Describe your dream for me! This might uncover the origin of your knee pain."*

I am so scared. That's when I usually wake up, sweating profusely and scared to death."

I begin to think that we are close to unraveling the mystery of her knee. I resolve to get to the heart of the issue by using the Gestalt therapy technique I outlined earlier. I will ask Allison to become each part of her dream, on the premise that each "actor," each "prop," and each "set" of the dream represents a different part of her personality and that ongoing conflicts among these different parts could be damaging her body. A common example of such a conflict would be a part of a person who loved her spouse pitted against a part that resented the same spouse for drinking too much.

In Allison's dream, besides herself, there are only four other elements: the car, the road, the emergency brakes, and the abyss. I ask Allison to become the car, first describing herself as the car.

She starts, "I am a very pretty small red Austin mini, and I am driving down a steep road."

At this juncture I think it is significant that she is describing her car self as a pretty red small car since Allison is a pretty short girl with red hair. There is a definite parallel there.

Allison is tense as she continues, "I have no more brakes. I'm going way too fast. I can't slow down. I'm going to crash."

As she talks, I can't help wondering: "Is Allison going too fast on the road of her life, something that only her unconscious can be aware of?" I know I should continue by asking her to become the road, but I decide to ask a different question:

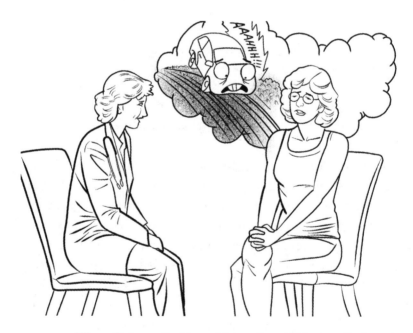

*Allison: "I dream that I am driving downhill in a car that*
*doesn't have any brakes!*
*I'm going to crash! I'm so scared!"*
*Doctor Chris: "Is anything in your life going too fast and scaring you?"*

"Allison, can what you just said be applied to the real Allison? Are you going too fast on the road of your real life?"

Allison seems surprised. "No, doc, everything is good . . . except . . ." She is deep in her thoughts.

Ah, the combination of her saying "except" and her being deep in her thoughts means her consciousness is accessing something important that has to be brought up to the surface.

I am eager to know. At first sight, a dream might have nothing to do with the symptom, but then, as the interpretation continues, a deep relationship can be uncovered.

"Except what?" I ask.

"Except that I am marrying Brad in two months." She looks very anxious.

Here, then, is the link. An upcoming wedding can be the source of deep anxiety.

At that point, my timer rings. It is time to remove her acupuncture needles. I pull them out and have her sit up. Her right knee is still hurting. Is there a relationship between her knee pain and her wedding in two months? Perhaps.

I go right to the heart of the matter. "Any parallel between the car being on a steep road without brakes and you getting married in two months?"

Allison moves into a very rigid posture. I notice a slight tremor in her jaw, and her right hand shakes a little. She seems to be struggling to say something but can't bring herself to do it. I also grow quiet and simply wait for her because I feel she is on the verge of an important insight. I don't want to say or do anything that will derail her. The wait is worth it. Suddenly, Allison bursts in tears. "Yes," she sobs. "The wedding is coming too fast. Brad wants to get married now! But I'm not sure I want to."

There is no doubt now that I have uncovered the reason for her recurring dream. Her conscious mind tells her to marry Brad in two months, and her unconscious mind tells her to not marry him so quickly—or maybe not marry him at all.

I decide to probe further and ask a question that very few primary care physicians would ask, "Maybe you don't want to marry him at all?"

Allison remains silent and sheds a few more tears. Her silence signals that I might be right.

It is now time to move deeper into Allison's issues, and for this I need her to give a voice to the road in her dream. I ask her first to describe herself as the road.

Allison dries her eyes, thinks a few seconds, then responds, "I am a narrow road, not very strong, and I am going directly into a dark abyss . . . Oh my God!" I take her exclamation to mean that she has suddenly realized that what she is describing could be applied to herself.

Yes, that is it! This is where the problem is. I decide to dive even deeper. "Do you love Brad?"

"I do, but he's always angry and puts me down all the time, especially when he has had too much to drink, and that happens more and more often." She looks sad.

I suddenly understand her unconscious mind. It probably knows that marrying Brad is a mistake. I have had several patients with a spouse suffering from alcohol addiction. Most of those marriages ended up in painful divorces. Her unconscious is perhaps foreseeing the future. Is her unconscious sending danger signals through the recurring dream? Through the knee pain?

My conversation with Allison shows that it is important to establish a deep human connection with a patient. Some people don't have anybody to confide in, and keeping inner struggles inside is sometimes destructive. The damage usually occurs in a weak body area as a consequence of unrelieved emotional stress. Sometimes a knee joint can suffer from chronic muscle tension or spasms in the quadriceps and/or hamstring muscles that flex and extend the knee. In addition, high levels of stress hormones such as cortisol can weaken the immune system and inhibit repair mechanisms of every day small injuries from muscle spasms.

Research on the connection between emotional suffering and knee pain has uncovered strong evidence of a link between emotional pain and knee pain. In Allison's case, it is possible that she hurt her knee when she was a child, thus weakening the joint and creating a vulnerable body part.

In any event, it is time to give her knee a voice.

Allison begins, "I am Allison's knee. I am usually healthy and strong but now I am hurting."

I ask, "Knee, what do you want Allison to do or not do?"

Allison "I don't want Allison to continue walking on me. I want her to stop going forward."

Allison suddenly realizes what she is saying. Indeed, her knee and her dream both seem to be suggesting that she has to stop moving forward in the direction her life is taking. It is not hard to speculate that her unconscious wants her to cancel the wedding.

Based on this insight, I now suspect that her knee pain results from constant tensing of all her muscles due to stress with a special emphasis on her right knee. I can only assume that she probably fell on it or twisted it when she was a child, which made it weaker than the other joints.

I discuss this possible diagnosis openly with Allison. She then leaves for home with her knee still hurting. But she has gained awareness of what her situation really is.

On the next weekend, Brad gets drunk and speaks to her angrily, insulting and humiliating her. She stands up to him and tells him she wants to cancel the wedding. Brad becomes violent, and Allison has to take refuge at her parents' house.

One month later, she and Brad are no longer together, and Allison's knee pain magically resolves.

Most symptoms will spontaneously resolve by themselves with little or no treatment when the stress causing them is removed. The fact that Allison's resolved after the breakup with Brad could be a simple coincidence or it could be directly related to the stress and muscle tension connection. There is no way to really know what happened.

My explanation is that her unconscious, knowing the wedding was a mistake, was making her body so tense that she was not walking in a relaxed, natural manner. As her feet hit the ground, with every step her legs became less flexible, had less range of motion, had less coordination between muscle groups, and had more tension. These actions hurt her knee joint.

A mechanical engineer named Mosche Feldenkrais developed a method based on physics and biomechanics for becoming more aware of our habitual neuromuscular patterns and rigidities and for expanding options for new ways of moving.

Applying his method, if you walk a few steps in slow motion with a relaxed mind, and then take few steps thinking about something stressful, you will notice that your way of walking will be completely different. Your feet will hit the ground very differently according to your state of mind. If you try this, you can understand how with chronic stress your joints could be hurting.

The consequence is that a person in pain will notice the physical pain and be unaware of the initial stressful origin of it. In Allison's case, her dream allowed us to shift that focus to her situation full of anxiety.

Although dream work produced quick, spectacular results for Allison, this Gestalt approach doesn't always enjoy the same easy success for two reasons.

First, not all physical problems have emotional roots, and not all patients' dreams lead to useful insights, even when emotional problems *are* the ultimate source of illness. Like any other method of diagnosis, dreams are sometimes revealing and sometimes not. It's not uncommon for me to spend an hour walking a patient through a dream, only to uncover nothing particularly useful.

Second, even when dreams *do* provide insights, it's often not easy to unravel their message, as was the situation with my patient Claudia.

Claudia's case is particularly interesting, not only because of the subtleties and complexities it presented, but also because it shows how to turn repressed negative emotions into conscious *positive* feelings.

Here is Claudia's story.

Claudia came to my office a few years ago for the first time, complaining of recurrent headaches that had started one year earlier. She was referred by her primary care physician who was out of treatment options.

As Claudia is talking about her headaches, I look at the X-rays she has placed on my desk. Her brain MRI is normal, and there is no problem with her sinuses. As for her dentist, he has given her a clean bill of health. I thought perhaps the problem might be in her cervical vertebrae, but cervical X-rays fail to show any abnormality. She says different treatments have helped her the last few months, but she has trouble tolerating them.

I pay attention to what she is wearing: high-heeled shoes, a black, knee-length dress, and a green and yellow blouse. Her hair is light brown and tied in a ponytail. She has applied some dark red lipstick to her thin lips. I look closely at her face. Her eyes look reddish and tired, and it is only 9:00 a.m.

Intrigued by her fatigued look, I ask her why she seems so tired. Her response is that she has been up since 4:00 a.m. because a dream woke her up. It seems like she might be still absorbed in her dream, since she tells me she has dreamt the same one many times.

Most physicians would not be interested in her dream, would ask more questions about her headaches, and would most likely conclude that she had a migraine condition. They would probably prescribe Sumatriptan.

But I am intrigued by her recurring dream. Her diagnosis probably *is* migraine headaches, but I am interested in the possible relationship between her recurrent headaches and her recurrent dream. I ask her to tell me about the dream.

Her face changes as she remembers it. I can see she is very worried. Her words come fast. Her body is shaking.

"Three men are pursuing me. I am running as fast as I can, but they are clearly running faster. I choose to get into a narrow street where lots of houses are wall to wall. One of them has a door slightly open. I push it open and close it after me, pressing my back against it, trying to calm my breathing down. Looking at the door, I see a lock which I quickly use. Maybe I am safe now. I hear heavy running footsteps from the road. They stop near my door. I hold my breath, hoping they won't hear my heart pounding in my chest. I hear male voices and footsteps move slowly away from me. I breathe deeply. I don't know why I am pursued, but I know I am in danger. Maybe I can find a phone to call the police. I explore the house. It is a big house with beautiful antique oak furniture in the living room. There doesn't seem to be anybody there."

As she speaks, I write down all the elements of the dream that I will urge her to give a voice to: three men, narrow street, house, door, lock, oak furniture. I think about stopping her, but she is so deeply into recounting her dream that I let her continue, deciding to enjoy her thrilling story.

"I suddenly realize I can call for help on my cell phone. I grab the purse I am carrying on my shoulder and open it. To my surprise, it is almost empty. My wallet and my cell phone are gone. Oh no! All my credit cards, my driver's license, cash, house and car keys, everything is gone! The only thing left in there is a red scarf."

I notice how shaken and distressed she looks and write down more elements of the dream: cell phone, purse, wallet, credit card, driver's license, cash, house and car keys, red scarf.

"Then I panic! When was everything stolen? How will I be able to fly back to California without money, ID, or credit card? How foolish I was to carry all my valuables with me. I should have left them in the hotel safe!!! Suddenly, I hear footsteps and male voices outside again. My heart pounds. I am so scared I am ready to scream! Voices are getting closer! They found where I'm hiding!!! Somebody is trying to open the front door, but they can't. Suddenly, I hear heavy banging. They are trying to force the door open. I have to hide. I look around in a panic, running everywhere, exploring the bedrooms. Where can I hide? My heart is thumping so hard it wakes me up."

Claudia is shaking and sweating profusely. I look at her more closely. I can see underarm sweat marks in the green and yellow silk fabric of her shirt. The rest of her dress is impeccable and shows her perfectly sculptured body. Her white, open-toed, high heels show her recently painted red toenails. Her light brown long hair in a ponytail is making her look younger than her forty six years. I am struck by the sharp contrast between her bright happy clothing and her sad and anxious looking face. What is really going on with her?

Can this recurring dream help us find the origin of the violent headaches she is experiencing every few days? Why did those headaches start one year ago? Did she have a problem at work, with her husband, or with her kids at that time?

As I ask her work- and family-related questions, possible origins of her headaches are eliminated one by one. Her job as a librarian is not stressful, and she is happily married with no children. I do find that other family members experience headaches. Her mother, who died of a sudden heart attack a year ago, did have occasional migraine headaches and her sister does too, but Claudia never used to have headaches before.

I have to find a different explanation. I ask her to give her headache a voice, but that doesn't get us anywhere.

I have a feeling that the answer is in her recurrent dream. Her subconscious is trying to give out clues, and she is not aware of them.

As I did with Allison, I want Claudia to give each part of the dream a voice. But there are so many parts of her dream. Where do I start? What part of her dream will give us the answer? I have to start somewhere, so I choose the house that she ran into. Usually, houses are a good choice because people easily understand how a house can be the symbol of self. I explain to Claudia that I want her to imagine she is the house in her dream and to describe it in the first person. She becomes the house.

Claudia begins, "I am a big house. I have elegant antique furnishings in me. I am old but kept in good shape."

She goes on a bit, but the house doesn't seem to be leading us anywhere. I ask her to switch and become the men pursuing her. In dream interpretation, when people are fighting other people, it is usually symbolic of two parts of the self fighting against each other. Revealing that inner conflict usually gives us meaningful results.

Claudia gets the hang of it. "I am those men pursuing Claudia and wanting to kill Claudia." Then, as Claudia, she says, "That doesn't make sense."

I reply, "We could interpret this as: 'There is a part of me that wants to kill another part of me.' What do you think?"

"Oh!" she exclaims. "So one part of me wants to kill another part of me, but that other part of me has to resist and stay alive. Yes, that's interesting!"

Now that she understands what we are getting at, I ask, "What parts of you want to kill other parts of you? And what part or parts of you do they want to kill?"

Claudia reflects for a moment, and then she says, "I am such a perfectionist, and it takes me so long to get things done the right way. Part of me wishes I were faster even if it meant I'd be messier. I would accomplish more, and my life would be much more fun if I was less of a perfectionist."

Is the inner conflict between her perfectionist self and her other self the source of her headaches? Possibly. Headaches often arise when someone is locked in an unconscious struggle with themselves. I say, "I suspect that your perfectionism may be triggering your headaches. Let's try an experiment for one week. Experiment with making things less perfect; for example, don't iron your clothes so perfectly, don't shine your shoes, leave more mess in your house before you leave for work, leave some dishes in the sink. At the library, leave work to be done the following day and see if your headaches decrease."

Claudia gulps. "Just thinking about doing things sloppily is very threatening to me."

I look at her a moment and ask, as gently as I can, "More threatening than the headaches?"

She takes a deep breath, nods, and leaves my office.

The following morning, I have a panicked phone call from her. She had the same dream again, and her headache, instead of decreasing, is getting worse. Her dream is so vivid and her headache so intense that I tell her to come in the office right away.

When she arrives, I note that she is wearing a blue shirt matching her blue jeans, that her hair is a mess, and that she has no make-up on. That is so unlike her—a clear sign that she is really shaken.

I ask her what part of last night's dream was so powerful. She says, "It was my purse! My credit cards, money, keys, glasses, makeup—everything was gone!"

It seems her unconscious is directing us towards her purse. What does it want to say? I need to ask her to try to give her purse a voice.

She responds immediately. "I am small but very strong. I am black, made with high quality leather. I usually contain every single thing that is important to Claudia. Everything that was valuable inside of me has suddenly disappeared. I am nothing anymore without those. I have no identity, no papers. I am stuck in Africa! I cannot travel and go back to the States. I cannot see clearly anymore because my glasses are gone. I cannot make myself beautiful because my makeup is gone. My priceless insides are gone. "Claudia's voice brakes and tears fill her eyes.

I suddenly remember a detail she had mentioned the day before. "Claudia," I say, "is there anything left in your purse? Anything at all?"

Claudia hesitates then after a few seconds, tells me, "Yes, this will sound really odd, but there is a red scarf."

In dream interpretation, when patients believe something about their dream is odd, that thing can have a deep meaning. Although psychiatrists and neuroscientists who study sleep and dreams have yet to unearth acceptable proof on the significance of specific events and symbols in dreams, many researchers believe that the research of Dr. Martin Seligman of the University of Pennsylvania comes close. His work suggests that the imagery of dreams very likely arises from "random neural processes," but a person's *interpretation* of those images is likely very meaningful.

Dr. Morton Reiser, a Yale psychiatrist, summed up this point of view when he observed, "The way the dreamer connects those elements gives them their meaning. That's how the mind exploits the brain in a dream. . . . Often what seems most obscure on the surface is what finally reveals a deeper meaning."

In my long experience working with dreams, I have learned to focus on images that stand out as being odd or out of place because I believe a patient's unconscious mind calls attention to images it wants the dreamer to be aware of specifically *by* making them appear weird or odd. For example, if you look at a photograph of a nature scene, your attention will not be drawn to any one element. But if the nature photograph randomly includes something that doesn't fit—like an airplane—your eye will immediate be drawn to the thing that doesn't fit.

I believe Claudia's unconscious knew this and "placed" the red scarf in her purse to call attention both to it and its deeper meaning.

I ask Claudia, "Talk as if you are that scarf. First describe it, then say everything that comes to mind. Don't censor yourself or hesitate."

Claudia begins, "I am red, long, made with premium quality silk. I bring warmth and comfort. I used to belong to Claudia's mother—" Claudia suddenly stops talking. She is softly crying.

I look at her intently. The fact that she is getting emotional when talking about her mother is, of course, meaningful. Are her headaches linked to her mother? I have noticed that a lot of people, even in their seventies, eighties, and older, still have a lot of emotions linked to their childhood. Some people are traumatized in their early years by their parents, never get over their traumas and suffer from the emotional consequences until the day they die. Some of those emotional consequences create medical symptoms and even illnesses. Is this true for Claudia?

"I am . . ." She stops again

"You are what?" I ask.

"I don't know, exactly. It's hard to put into words."

"Then stop thinking about it, and tell me the first thing that pops into your head."

Claudia hesitates "Well, this is going to sound weird, but the first words that come to me are . . . umbilical cord." Her look of puzzlement is quickly followed by a sharp intake of breath. She begins to sob quietly.

I have very mixed feelings about this new development. Part of me wants to hold on to my insight that the conflict between perfectionist Claudia and "normal" Claudia is causing her headaches. But when I see how deeply affected Claudia is by the death of her mother, I realize perfectionism might not be the only cause—or even the biggest cause—of Claudia's problem. Her umbilical cord allusion strengthens this conclusion. Our unconscious, which often knows the deep truth about the source of our troubles, tries hard to communicate with our conscious mind whenever we have severe chronic stress. In earlier chapters I explained how our unconscious tries to get our attention through physical symptoms such as skin rashes, knee pain and belly pain.

The unconscious has other ways of communicating with us. Images, such as the red scarf are one of these ways, and seemingly random words, such as umbilical cord, are another.

As I mentioned, whenever strange or random images, words, or songs come into our head, our unconscious—which doesn't communicate in linear, logical sentences—is trying to tell us something.

But Claudia's unconscious isn't subtly suggesting that she pay attention to her mother. It is screaming for her to pay attention to her mother.

I lightly place my hand on her shoulder and in a low voice I ask, "Do you miss your mother?"

As she nods yes, I realize that if I continue on this road, I run the risk of having her spiral downward emotionally. She might start focusing on how much she misses her mom. Possibly she could become more depressed and even sink into deep depression. Instead, I need to *turn her repressed negative emotion of loss into a positive healing emotion of love and closure.*

I decide to have her focus on the conversation she would like to have with her mom if she could. I grab the chair that was against the wall and place it in front of her. Then I choose a white pillow from the pile of pillows in the corner of the room and place it on the chair saying, "Let's pretend your mom is this white pillow and can hear you. Is there anything you would like to tell her?"

Claudia composes herself and shakes her head. Then grabs the white pillow, goes to the pillow pile in the corner of the room, throws the white pillow on top of the pile, and grabs a red pillow and places it on the chair across from her. "She liked red!"

After taking a few deep breaths, she reaches in front of her to touch the red pillow and begins to speak. "Mom, I miss you. It's been a year. I am sorry, I didn't have time to say goodbye to you. Your heart attack took you so suddenly." She looks at me, her eyes filled with tears.

I am very touched by what she is saying and the way she is touching the red pillow, but what strikes me is the timing of all this. She just indicated that her mom had her heart attack a year before our session, which is when Claudia's headaches started. This is an important clue.

I need to push deeper. "What else would you like to tell your mom?"

Claudia becomes very emotional. "I want to tell you, Mom, how much I love you. I am so thankful you gave me this wonderful life. I criticized you sometimes, but I know you did the best you could, as a single mom, in raising me and my sister. I never did openly thank you, and I regret that! I never did openly tell you I loved you and I regret that. I should have told you, then. . . . So, I am telling you now, hoping you can hear me." She pauses, sobbing.

This is a proper goodbye. This is real closure. I am glad she is able to do this since this closure may improve her health through decreasing her inner turmoil.

After calming down, she continues talking to the red pillow. "Thank you for all the unconditional love you gave me! Thank you for raising me the way you did! I love you so much!!!" She pauses and crying again, manages to say, "Thank you for giving me the gorgeous red scarf!" She stops.

This red scarf is definitely the clue to solving Claudia's problem. This means there is one more thing left to do. I must move Claudia toward saying a final goodbye to her mother. There are different ways to do this. I have found that the most effective way is through visual effects, one of them being to have the patient physically and symbolically "cut the umbilical cord."

Neuroscientists and psychologists have shown why performing a physical action works so well. We understand our own motivations and emotions the same way we understand them in others—by observing behavior. When we observe ourselves performing a physical act, such as cutting an umbilical cord, our brain, in its never-ending quest to make sense of the world, constructs a narrative after the fact that says, "I must feel this way because I just *behaved this way*."

So I say to Claudia, "In order for your life to start again fresh, I need you to cut the umbilical cord. Let's pretend there is an imaginary red scarf going from the red pillow to you. Continue saying what you need to say to your mom, and when you are ready, take two fingers, pretend they are scissors, say goodbye, and cut the imaginary red scarf."

Claudia continues talking for a while, and then, trembling, moves the index and middle finger of her right hand up in a gesture of cutting and severs the imaginary red scarf that represents the umbilical cord. Claudia is still touching the red pillow with her left hand.

It is a very emotional and beautiful moment. A torrent of tears flows from my eyes. I am suddenly taken back in time and begin to think about my attachment to my dad. I am struggling with strong feelings tied to our relationship and his passing. But being the physician, I am not supposed to show my own emotions in front of a patient. I try to repress my tears and avoid Claudia's gaze so that she wouldn't see my eyes. But I can't. I decide to be bluntly honest and not try to hide my own feelings. I am a doctor, but also a human being very touched by her session.

She sees my raw emotion and seems to be very touched by it. I am afraid this will alter her experience, but it doesn't appear to. As a matter of fact, she seems encouraged by my empathy.

After taking a few deep breaths, she says, "Bye, Mom" and slowly removes her hand from the red pillow.

She remains silent for a while. I respect her silence, take a few deep breaths myself, and look at her intently. She seems calm and serene now, perhaps at peace.

After what seems like a long time but is probably just a few seconds, I ask, "How is your headache now?"

She looks at me with surprise, suddenly remembering why she is here. "It's much better! I don't feel the throbbing pain in my forehead and behind my eyes anymore. Maybe this is what my body needed! Closure! Thank you so much!"

As Claudia leaves my office, I wonder whether her headaches are really related to her mom. This need for closure might just be a coincidence. In any case, what I am sure of is that the closure was unconsciously acutely needed and that what just happened will make her stronger.

That night, I cannot fall asleep, tossing and turning, thinking about Claudia's case and remembering my dad. It has been fifteen years since he passed away, but I feel the need to connect with him again. At 1:00 a.m., I finally decide to get up, go to my living room, grab two pillows—a brown one and a purple one—and place them both on the carpet facing each other. I sit on the purple one (one of my favorite colors).

Imagining my dad is the brown pillow because he often wore brown clothes, I tell him how thankful I am for the positive way he influenced my life. He showed me what it takes to be a good person and a great physician (he was a physician himself). I tell him how many fond memories I have of him and how much I love him.

When I finish talking to him, I switch seats and sit on the brown pillow, imagining it is my dad now talking to me, telling me how much he loves me too.

Moving back to my purple seat, I take a deep breath and inhale all the love I just received. Then, smiling, I go back to bed and quickly fall fast asleep.

Two weeks later, I have a surprise visit from Claudia. She has with her a beautiful light purple orchid plant in full bloom and a thank you note. Her recurring dream has not come back, and her headaches have decreased in intensity to the point that they are now very manageable without drugs.

Claudia's improvement clearly shows that I made the right decision in focusing on her dream and directing her to say goodbye to her mother. It is critically important to have closure with people who are dear to us. I have seen many people become depressed, fatigued, and suffer emotionally and physically because they didn't have the opportunity to say goodbye to a dying parent, to a mate, or other loved one.

Once depression sets in, elevated stress hormones such as Cortisol depress the immune system and people have more trouble fighting infections or even diseases like cancer. Those patients come to my office multiple times for numerous illnesses ranging from bronchitis to sinus infection to headaches to indigestion due to overeating, and other sickness. If they have any small pain anywhere, it is experienced as a much stronger pain because of the depression, which makes people even more depressed, and which makes them experience even more pain—all of which becomes a vicious circle.

I can think of several possible explanations for her lack of closure bringing on severe headaches: One is that it triggered muscle tensions and spasms all over her body, but particularly on weaker parts around her neck. Another explanation is that intense headaches like Claudia's can arise from heightened response to pain signals in parts of the brain dealing with emotions. Many people experience discomfort in and around the head, but those with anxiety, depression, and other emotional problems have a much greater conscious *awareness* of the pain.

I hope I have shown you how very meaningful dreams can be and how they can be a gateway for healing. Of course, in practicing this way, I become more deeply involved in my patients' lives than most internists do. But that is what I love about my work. I learn about their everyday lives. I witness their sadness, hope, anger, happiness, and more. I see how their emotions influence their symptoms and vice versa. And most of all, I get to make a very positive impact on their lives.

## A Healing-Secret Exercise

*Here's a practical exercise to use with your dreams.*

Always keep a piece of paper and a pen by your bedside.

If you wake up at night in the middle of a dream, immediately grab that pen and write down what your dream is about. Write down every single detail about your dream. Describe the people and also the objects in your dream.

Describe how you feel.

If one object looks odd or out of place, pay special attention to it and describe it even more precisely.

You have to do this before you get up to go to the bathroom. If you can't wait and go to the bathroom before writing your dream down, chances are that most of your memory of it will be flushed down the toilet. By the time you get back into bed, your dream will be forgotten.

In the morning, read your notes, and give a voice to each element of the dream in the first person. For example: I am a red car, I am small, I am used for ___. Or I am a clock (if there is a clock in your dreams), I am used for ____ etc.

Also, describe the emotion you were feeling in your dream. See if it correlates with any current emotion in your life.

If you have an illness or a pain anywhere, see if what you are saying correlates with a possible origin of your symptom.

Keep an open mind and you'll learn a great deal about yourself, about your unconscious, and about your body.

# 7

# Conversations in Nature

I TAKE HOUR-LONG NATURE walks with patients. I don't do it for exercise, although it is good exercise. I do it because walking in nature is one of my healing secrets. It helps me diagnose and treat certain of my patients' medical problems. I take this highly unconventional approach to medicine whenever I am convinced that the root cause of the presenting symptoms is emotional, and that other techniques that I've described thus far in the book don't work at first.

For example, I have noticed that sometimes, in cases of depression, chronic fatigue syndrome, or chronic muscle pain, the origin of the disease is so deeply buried inside the unconscious that it is difficult to access it, even when I try to access it directly by giving voice to the body. Yet locating the real origin of the disease is key for a long lasting cure.

In cases that don't respond, I need to use one of my indirect tools. We already saw how I use dream interpretation. That's one of my indirect tools. The other, addressed in this chapter, is taking my patient out for a walk!

It's not just any walk, it's a special walk in nature.

By going out on a nature walk with my patients, I become more of a friend and confident. I find that I am able to probe their deeper self via the "back door," which is much less protected than the "front door" and allows me to bypass defense mechanisms. I call the "back door" the door to the body via the unconscious. I call the "front door" the door to the body via consciousness.

By leaving the office with my patient, I also decrease the risk of the patient exhibiting white coat syndrome. That's what happens when patients are intimidated by doctors in their white coats and become very tense and defended.

Once we are outside and in nature, my belief is that whatever my patient's eyes are drawn to is related to what he or she is unconsciously and deeply experiencing.

This belief is supported by many psychologists and behavioral researchers who have discovered that many of our thoughts, emotions, and behaviors are not random, but originate in our unconscious. So I believe that the things my patients might casually notice on walks are not really random thoughts; these choices of what is observed are governed by unconscious processes and are meaningful.

In other words, there is a reason we see what we see, notice what we notice.

During a walk in a park not far from my office with my patient Mark, I ask him what is catching his eyes. He says, "I love clouds, but I am drawn to this tree, far away, the brown one. For some reason, I can't take my eyes off it."

What brown tree? I don't see it. I look where he is pointing. I can see a lot of tall green trees but no brown tree. Looking more attentively, in the middle of the green trees is indeed a brown tree that looks in really bad shape. I would have never noticed it if Mark hadn't told me about it. This is interesting.

I would have picked one of the green trees, a flower, or a bird. However, Mark focused on a brown sick-looking tree. Why? His choice tells me that, at this moment at least, he is consciously or unconsciously seeing himself as this old, dying brown tree.

Why am I strolling in the park with Mark? No, it's not a botany walk. I am trying to figure out what is happening to him.

Mark's aunt, a long-time patient, has sent him to me, saying that he is always tired and seems depressed. She is hoping I can help him.

When he arrives in my office for the first time one week before our walk, I am immediately impressed by his strikingly blue eyes and his serious demeanor in contrast to his very casual clothing and baseball hat. His tall stature and slim figure are pleasant to the eye. He quickly glances at me, and then, looking down, he shakes my hand. His grasp is very soft and his hand big and sweaty.

I am already puzzled by the contrast between his strong appearance and his weak hand shake. Also, his sweaty hands can mean he is feeling stressed. But most of all, the fact that he only looks at me directly in the eye for a split second and shakes my hand without looking at me means, in my experience, that part of him is hiding and doesn't want to be seen.

I pay attention to what he is wearing: a white, worn out t-shirt, pale green shorts, and tennis shoes that have seen better days, all of which makes me think he doesn't have much money.

He sits down in the chair I point at opposite me, arms crossed in front of him, legs crossed in a clearly protective posture.

Alright, I already know he is so guarded that it will be a difficult case to solve.

"Mark, welcome to my office! Tell me, how old are you?"

"Twenty," he replies in a harsh voice. He still does not look at me directly. Instead he is gazing out the window with its view of the picturesque town in which my office is located. I follow his glance. The sky is blue, and the view is clear that Friday morning in July. There is no fog and it looks like the day is going to be beautiful and warm, just the kind of weather I like. Mark seems to like the outdoors. He doesn't seem to really want to be in my office, which is often the case when young people are referred to me by a family member. But since he is here, I want to do the best I can to help, even if it isn't much.

I hesitate between launching into some small talk in the hope that he will let his guard down or taking a direct approach. I have a feeling he is so guarded that either way won't make a difference. I choose the direct approach.

"Your aunt wanted me to see you. She says you are very tired every day and can't sleep well at night. Is that true?"

Mark glances quickly at me then shifts his eyes back to the window. "Yes, but nobody can help me."

"Why do you say that? Maybe I can help you. Would you be willing to try something fun and new?"

Mark looks at me directly for the first time. The darkness I see there is striking. A thought comes to my mind: Could he be depressed? I look at his arms, which are still crossed against his body, as he answers. "Sure."

I explain that I want him to imagine his body could have a voice and could talk out loud. "What does your body have to say?"

Mark doesn't hesitate. In a monotone he says, "I am tired."

I try to probe further, but I can't get any useful or precise answers from his body's voice. I decide to try something else and ask him to take a couple of deep breaths, relax, and then be aware of his body. I ask if any part of his body is bothering him at the moment. But he says nothing is bothering him.

I decide to examine him and look at the blood work his primary care physician did. Everything looks within normal range.

Now I am convinced that his fatigue is connected somehow with his unconscious. None of my direct approaches are working, so it is time to try an indirect one. Since he seems transfixed by the view from my office window, I ask him if he likes walking in nature. Uncrossing his arms for the first time, he replies that he does. I then offer to go with him for a walk in a nearby park the following morning at 8:00 am.

Mark's expression changes. I can see both surprise and an intense sadness in his beautiful blue eyes. "I have never gone for a walk with a doc as part as an office visit. This is strange."

I smile "I like to surprise people! So, see you tomorrow morning at eight o'clock at the corner entrance to the park nearest my office."

As he leaves, I decide to ask his aunt about his background, his childhood, his life story.

When we speak by phone later that day, she tells me Mark had a difficult childhood. He was constantly fighting and arguing with his parents. He wouldn't do household chores like washing the dishes or taking out the trash. He didn't get along with his younger brother, either. The brother was five years younger than Mark and a much more obedient child. He did everything his parents asked and never fought with them. As a result, he got along with them very well, earning their praise and gratitude.

Academically, Mark did well. He had been an A student all his life, graduated from high school with honors, was accepted by USC, and began to attend as a business administration major.

Halfway through his first year of college, his parents died in a car accident. His aunt took Mark and his brother into her home.

Understandably, that's when the problems started. He began waking up at two o'clock in the morning unable to go back to sleep. Even when he would go to bed at 11:00 p.m., he would wake up at 2:00 a.m. As a result, he was extremely tired during the day and not able to concentrate. One month later, unfortunately, he dropped out of college and took a job as a counter clerk at McDonald's.

His aunt became very worried and took him to her primary care physician who ran a battery of tests, all of which were normal. The doctor recommended he see a psychiatrist. The psychiatrist put him on antidepressants, which made him feel even worse.

Taking the antidepressants, Mark became so tired that he missed several of his shifts at McDonald's and was fired. The psychiatrist told him to continue taking the antidepressants for at least one month, as sometimes they take that long to work. As the month progressed, Mark became increasingly fatigued. Continually exhausted, he stayed in bed for longer and longer hours. On day twenty-four, he decided on his own to stop the treatment. He refused to go back to the psychiatrist.

His aunt, more and more worried, knew that I had cured her best friend of her chronic fatigue syndrome, so she made an appointment for Mark to see me.

At that time, it had been thirteen months since his parents had died.

Mark's aunt and I finish speaking. As I hang up the phone, I reflect on how terrible it must have been for Mark to lose his parents. Usually people who lose a loved one begin to feel progressively better after six months. But it's been over a year for Mark, and he is getting worse.

The following day is a Saturday. I wake up energized knowing I will start my day with a walk in the park with Mark. He is on time, wearing the exact same shorts, tennis shoes, and baseball hat he had on yesterday. Well at least he changed the t-shirt. It's black this time. He hasn't shaved, and the look suits him well.

I ask about his night, hoping he had a dream I could use as an indirect way of getting to his unconscious. Unfortunately, he doesn't remember dreaming. He does say that he didn't sleep well, woke up at 2:00 a.m., and is exhausted. Undoubtedly his unconscious is worried about something.

In order to learn more, I need to lower his defenses with some casual conversation. Then I plan to ask him a seemingly innocuous question about what he is looking at, or rather what are his eyes being drawn to in the park. Once I have him focusing on an element of nature, I plan on having him talk as if he is this bit of nature, whatever it may be. These tactics should move him outside of his body and allow me to gather good information about his unconscious.

After a few minutes of talking about the heavy metal music he enjoys and the baseball teams he follows, he seems to relax. He is ready for the next step.

As we continue walking at a slow pace, I look around. The park is beautiful, with a view of the ocean off in the distance; the weather is sunny with light white clouds in the sky. We can even see small ocean waves crashing against the shoreline. I can see red, yellow, and purple flowers with humming birds hovering around them. I can see tall, majestic blooming trees. The whole scene is beautiful, and there is much to notice and admire all around us. There are a lot of various elements to choose from in the surrounding scenery. I am curious as to what Mark will be drawn to.

I ask *the* question: "Mark, when you look at this scenery around us, the sky, the ocean, the flowers, the birds, the trees, is there anything that catches your eye, anything that stands out and attracts your gaze, anything that you want to spend time looking at?"

After taking a few seconds to look around, Mark focuses on the only brown, sickly tree in the middle of all that beautiful green. Strange choice, I am thinking. This tree looks dead to me. It's not a thing I, or most people, would want to gaze at. I need to ask him to describe this tree—the way it appears to him. I hope his defenses are now down.

Mark seems, for a change, to be relaxed. "This tree looks like it's a dead tree, or if it isn't dead, it's dying. It has a couple of green leaves, but the rest is pretty much dead."

My thoughts are confirmed: He too sees death in the tree he has chosen. I notice that Mark himself is bringing up the concept of death and dying in association with the tree. He is telling me that part of him is dying. But it is too soon to ask him if or how the concept of death relates to him. I cannot take the risk of his defensiveness taking control again. First, I need to learn more. I do this by asking him to tell me about the different parts of the tree.

I ask about the tree roots, significant because they might serve as a symbol of the deeper part of Mark. He answers the way I am afraid he might. "I think they are pretty dead too."

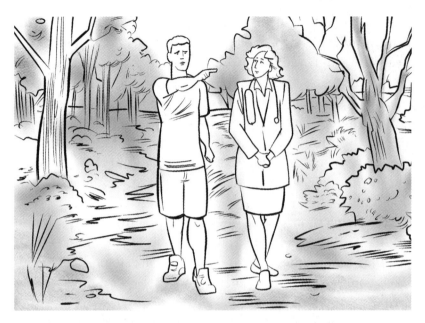

*Doctor Chris: "Let's explore why you are feeling fatigued and depressed!
Does anything in this scenery grab your attention?"
Mark: "That brown tree grabs my attention!"
Doctor Chris: "Can you talk as if you were that tree?"*

I want to keep Mark's guard down and at the same time learn more about his unconscious. I do so by keeping him focused on his tree and its roots with questions to stimulate his imagination. "Why is this tree and its roots dying? Can you imagine a story explaining this?" The first thing that comes to his mind is probably most tightly related to what his unconscious is experiencing.

After a few seconds of silence, he responds, "It could have been poisoned."

Now I need to probe deeper with a question I hope will seem superficial to him. "What story comes to mind on how the tree was poisoned?"

Mark reflects for what seems like a full minute. "It is poisoned everyday by somebody who comes at night and pours a deadly mixture on its roots. It has been going on for quite a while. A few more months like this and it will be completely dead."

Wow. Here is a connection to Mark's health. I interpret it as Mark himself being "poisoned" every day. That would explain his intense fatigue. I probe deeper. "Do you think the tree can be saved?"

"I don't know," he replies.

"Let's say you knew the answer. If you knew, what would you say?"

"The tree might still be saved because there are still some healthy leaves on some of the branches, but anyone who wants to save it shouldn't wait too long."

I now know enough. It is time to bring his tree story closer to home. I ask him to talk as if he were the tree, using the first person. By doing this, I run the risk of having his guard coming back up, but I must take the chance, for his sake.

Mark is reluctant at first but then finally responds. "Well, I guess I must be this brown tree. I only have a couple of green leaves left on me. I am dying." He pauses.

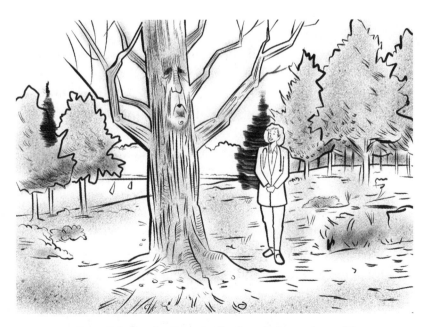

*Tree: "I feel so bad! Looks like I am being poisoned!"*

Gently, I urge him to go on.

"I used to be thriving. Once upon a time I was this beautiful sturdy tree with strong roots. Everybody admired me, but somebody started watering my roots with poison every evening, and it is destroying me little by little. There is not much life left in me. Soon I'll be completely dead."

Mark's voice suddenly weakens as he realizes the purpose of the exercise and the relevance to his own life. He lets out a quiet moan and stops walking.

It is now time for me to take the direct approach, risky because he may resist and the moment will be gone.

"Are you dying Mark? Is anybody poisoning you every evening?"

Mark stays silent. I've touched a sensitive point. Is he going to close up and stop talking? I decide to wait in silence. Fortunately, after a few seconds, he continues, "I get depressed at night so I go to my car and drink whiskey and eat potato chips that I hide there."

"How much whiskey?"

Mark "Two or three shots."

This is it! Mark is finally opening up! Our walk in nature is working.

Whiskey every night could explain why he is more depressed. Alcohol can worsen mood. It could also cause or worsen sleep apnea, especially if Mark sleeps on his back, which I confirm by asking him. His tongue probably slides backwards and obstructs his airway during sleep making him suffocate several times an hour when he breathes in. Good quality sleep becomes impossible and fatigue the next day, along with deepening depression follow. I have all the pieces of my puzzle except for one.

Why does Mark need to drink whiskey at night? Is it because he misses his parents or is there a deeper, more complex problem? I simply go ahead and ask him.

His brow furrows, and he replies, "Because if I don't drink, I have thoughts."

"What kind of thoughts?"

Mark now looks at the ground. "Guilty thoughts."

This must be the missing piece. What is he feeling guilty about? Did he commit any crime? Or could he be feeling guilty for his parents' death? I have seen this in the past: When parents divorce or die, some children think it is their fault even though they are blameless. The belief is destructive and can create depression and chronic fatigue. Sometimes the problem is never addressed over a lifetime. I have seen patients in their seventies still suffering acutely from childhood issues which cause physical symptoms difficult to treat with conventional medications. The sooner such problems are addressed, the better.

It seems that Mark is now willing to open up and stay open to my questions. I decide to continue with my direct approach.

"What are you feeling guilty about? Is this related to your parents' death?"

Mark answers in a barely audible voice. "Yes."

"How? How is it related?"

Mark starts walking towards the dying tree. Keeping pace, I walk next to him. He remains silent for a time, then begins speaking softly. "I always argued with them! That day, we had a huge argument. They asked me to clean my room. I told them it was my room and I could do anything I wanted with it. They told me it was their house, so I needed to obey their rules. I got very angry and told them I was going to leave *their* house for good that night and that they would never see me again. I don't know if they believed me or not. But we avoided each other for the rest of the day. Later on they left in the car for dinner. That's when the accident happened . . . they died because of me . . .

We have arrived at the tree. Mark suddenly breaks down and sits on the ground under the dying tree, sobbing. I sit down next to him. Everything makes sense now. I understand his guilt, his depression, his lack of sleep, his fatigue. As a confidant, as well as his physician, I am feeling his pain acutely and am sad for him. But I am his doctor, and most of all I need to help him. How can I get him out of this vicious circle? I could refer him to a psychotherapist, but will he go and will he open up? Will another treatment of antidepressants help?

I could offer medications, but the problem is buried so deep in Mark that they will not be very effective. Despite the fact that about one in ten Americans take antidepressants, the drugs are sometimes only slightly better than placebos (sugar pills), and those people that *do* benefit from antidepressants often experience only partial relief from their symptoms. But there are many side effects to these drugs, and they are very common. They include fatigue, constipation, appetite changes, and sexual dysfunction. So in my opinion the risks outweigh the possible benefits, especially since the drugs hadn't helped him previously.

Mark's case shows why it is so important to find the deep cause of an illness rather than just using drugs as a bandage. Drugs are most likely not going to cure someone whose has deep-rooted, unresolved emotional conflicts such as Mark's.

I dismiss the idea of drugs. Mark is opening up to me right now. I have the opportunity right now, under this tree, to start bringing him back to health.

I decide to start by using reason to help him understand that he did not cause the accident. "I get that you feel guilty, but in reality, the accident isn't your fault. Your parents happened to be in the wrong place at the wrong time."

Mark doesn't buy it. "They probably were thinking about what I said to them, that l was leaving, and they weren't paying attention to the road. I *know* I am responsible for their death."

"So, now, because of what happened, you are killing yourself slowly with whiskey every night? Is this what your parents would have wanted? Do you think they would say, "Mark, our son, we want you to die?"

Mark almost whispering, replies, "No."

My next step is critical.

In similar situations I have arranged an imaginary dialogue between the deceased person and the patient so that the issue can be seen from a new perspective—that of the deceased person. The technique often resolves the issue. I need to bring in the perspective of Mark's parents in a way that he can hear and accept.

I grab a few large brown leaves from the ground and make two piles touching each other. (If we were in my office, I would have used two pillows.) "Let's imagine that these leaves represent your parents. Let's imagine you can talk to them and they can talk to you. Tell your parents how you feel."

Mark is very surprised by my request and reluctant at first to go along with it. But he seems to have decided to trust me, and soon he begins to speak. "Mom and Dad, I wish you were still alive! I feel so bad! I am so sorry I had that argument with you. If I hadn't argued with you, you would probably still be alive." Mark is sobbing.

I need Mark's continued trust for the next step, which is to have him switch places and roles with the leaves, become his parents, and respond to Mark. It's a difficult switch that takes courage. When I ask him if he would now imagine what his parents would say to him, he at first, shakes his head. But a few minutes later, he gets up and carefully sits on the piles of leaves across from him.

I see his face and body change as if getting into character. His back was slumped but now becomes straight; his face becomes hard and serious as I imagine his parents were.

I ask quietly, "Are you Mark's mom or Mark's dad?"

Mark's voice is lower and sounds older and more mature. Looking at me, he answers, "I am Mark's dad." Then looking at where Mark had been sitting, he addresses Mark. "You were a bad son, never helping out, never doing the chores we asked you to do, never cleaning your room or helping with dishes or trash, always arguing with us." He pauses.

I decide to ask Mark's dad a key question. "Do you think it is Mark's fault that you got into a car accident? You can see that he is slowly killing himself now because of his guilt. What do you think about that?"

Mark, speaking as his father, does not hesitate. "No, it isn't his fault at all. He had nothing do with our accident. It just happened! A truck ran a red light and slammed into us. No one but that truck driver is to blame for our deaths." He continues, "Son, we don't want you to kill yourself because of that. We gave you life. We want you to enjoy it fully!"

I jump in. "Thank you, Mark's dad! Is there anything else you want to tell Mark?"

Mark continues in his dad's voice "We love you very much, son."

I decide to have Mark get up and switch places again and sit next to me in his original spot. I remind him of what was just said. "Did you hear what your father said? Your parents love you. Your dad says the accident wasn't your fault. You shouldn't destroy yourself because of this. Your parents gave you life. Your life is one of their most precious achievements. They want you to enjoy it and be happy."

Mark looks stunned, but he manages to say, "Yes, I think you're right!"

I continue in a kind but firm voice. "You need to stop drinking alcohol and start living. How about we get you in a bereavement group where you can spend some time processing and understanding all this? Are you willing?"

Mark is almost smiling. "Yes, Doc." His facial expression is completely changed. He seems relieved, and I can see that hope is alive in him. He seems now to want to find his way back to health. I believe he will do as I ask.

Before we go our separate ways, I instruct him to start sleeping on his side and, since when I ask him if he wants to attend a detox treatment center, he says he doesn't want to, I ask him if he is willing to decrease his alcohol intake to only one shot of whiskey a night. In that way he will at least cut down his alcohol consumption immediately. He agrees to try this. I offer to see him in my office the following Friday, and he accepts.

The following week when he arrives for his session, he looks so much better. He is open with me, telling me that he is feeling less guilty, sleeps better, is less fatigued, and in a better frame of mind. We have stopped the vicious circle of guilt, alcohol, insomnia, fatigue, depression. Now he has a way to regain his health and his life.

I continue seeing Mark in my office every week. He eventually stops drinking completely and feels well enough to go back to college.

I hear later that Mark joined a bereavement group and remained with it for six months. It worked for him. He stayed in college and even earned an MBA with honors.

A walk in nature helped my patient step outside his body, and it allowed me to make a difficult diagnosis and clear up a deep emotional problem that might have eventually cost Mark his life.

It is amazing to me how, when I take different patients on this same walk on the same paths, with the same flowers, trees, shrubs in view, they choose completely different natural elements of the park to identify with. When I take another of my patients, Wendy, on the same walk, she focuses on a colorful butterfly that flutters past her. By giving that butterfly a voice, she is able to locate the origin of her shoulder pain and uncover a suppressed emotional need to visit far-away friends that she sorely missed.

Wendy's choice is so different and far less dramatic and melancholic than a dying tree, but just as important for the health of my patient. We all see things, and perhaps need to see things, differently.

## Healing-Secret Exercises

*Here's a practical exercise in observing nature:*

Pay close attention to your surroundings on your next walk.

Look attentively at what you are seeing, including the sky, clouds, trees, flowers, animals, insects, and the ground.

Choose a particular animate or inanimate object that you sense you are drawn to.

First focus on it and describe it.

Then become that object and speak as though it were you.

If you listen carefully to what you are saying, you will learn something new about yourself and your body.

*Here's anther practical exercise to help with grief at death of a loved one:*

Is there unfinished business between you and someone who is now dead?

If there is, choose two pillows of different colors: one for you and one for that someone who has passed away.

Place the two pillows on the floor facing each other.

Sit on the one representing you, and tell the other person what you always wanted to say.

When you have finished telling the person everything you want to say, get up and sit on the other pillow that represents the other person.

Imagine what the person would tell you in response.

Then go back to your pillow and reply to the person.

Do as many back and forth conversations as you wish.

Expressing aloud what has never been possible before is very cathartic and therapeutic.

It will give you a deep satisfaction, and this deep feeling will improve your health.

# 8

# A Drawing Worth
# Ten Thousand Words

THIS IS A drawing that I created to replicate one that an adult
patient drew for me to illustrate his feelings in childhood. I
am using it here as an example of how I am able to use a patient's
imagery to discover the origins of a patient's afflictions and eliminate them. The composite patient in my example is an eight-
year-old boy called Michael.

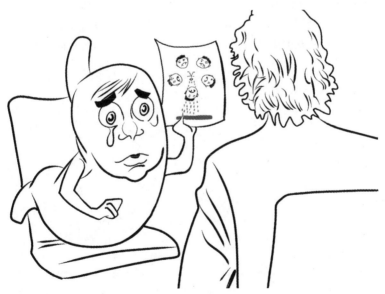

*If my stomach could draw, this is what it would make.*

Not all of us can give our bodies a voice. Sometimes patients are unable or unwilling to do so. With some patients, especially children, my preferred technique for getting to the deep origins of their illnesses is the use of art, and most often their drawings.

Dr. Cathy Malchiodi, a pioneering child therapist, points out that expressing our emotions is difficult even for adults. But kids, especially young ones, simply don't have the words to express what they are feeling. So creating artwork might be the only way to reach them.

Like walking in nature, the creation of art under my direction bypasses inner defenses that even children develop at a very young age. By asking my patient to focus on making a drawing and commenting on it, the door to his unconscious opens, allowing seemingly meaningless colors and shapes to express in free flowing manner some deeply buried emotions.

It has long been known that art expresses feelings. Some very famous painters created emotion-drenched work as a way to express their deep selves. Vincent van Gogh (1853–1890) is a great example. He was prone to extreme depression and epileptic seizures. In a 1889 self-portrait he conveys the strong emotions that appear to be swirling around the artist. You can see the intensity revealed in his eyes.

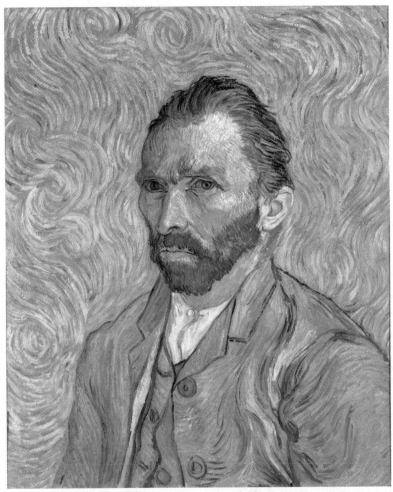

*Vincent Van Gogh* Portrait de l'artiste *painted in 1889*

In a painting called *Sorrowing Old Man* Van Gogh conveys that he clearly understood despair!

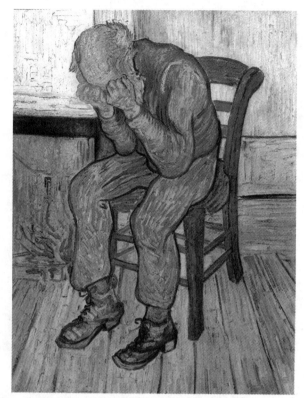

Sorrowing Old Man *painted by Vincent Van Gogh in 1890*

Van Gogh's good friend Paul Gauguin (1848–1903) also had severe bouts of debilitating depression and expressed his emotions through painting, sculpting, ceramics, prints, and other works. In Gauguin's self-portrait you can see his intensity and imagine his feelings about the suffering shown on his painting of Christ behind him.

Gauguin was involved in the development of the French Post-Impressionist movement, as well as in the development of Symbolism, an artistic and poetic movement using symbolic images and indirect suggestion to express emotions and states of mind.

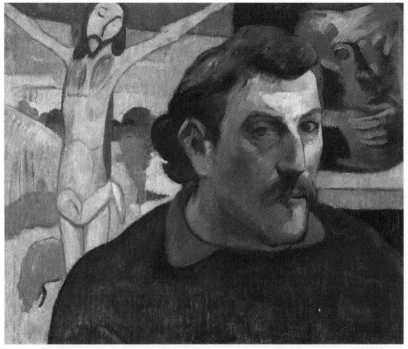

*Paul Gauguin's* Portrait of the Artist with the Yellow Christ,
*painted in 1899*

Painting and drawing are frequently used by individuals on their own, or in therapy, as a way of coping with a stressful situation, but they are rarely used by physicians to help make a diagnosis of a physical illness.

But I have found that in some cases, it can be extremely useful and allows for both diagnosis and treatment and a long lasting cure, as we'll see in Michael's story.

Michael, his sister Sarah, and their single mom, Rachel, had been patients of mine for several years when they lived in Los Angeles. When they moved to New York, Rachel had trouble finding a physician she liked so she continued calling me for simple health problems.

During one call, she told me about Michael's belly pain. It had been on and off for three weeks, and she was worried.

It just so happened that at the time of her call, I was about to fly to Paris to visit my mother. I decided to stop over in New York for a couple of days in order to examine Michael. Rachel offered to put me up at her place, and I gladly accepted. It had been a year since I had seen Rachel or the kids, and I was looking forward to visiting them.

I land in New York on a Tuesday night and make my way to the family's fourth floor apartment in an upscale building in Queens. When I arrive, I am welcomed by an energetic eleven-year-old, Sarah. She looks like a young woman already with long slightly auburn hair and hazel eyes surrounded by long dark eyelashes. She has grown a lot since last time I saw her. Her tight pink t-shirt shows budding breasts. Her dark purple skirt is fitting her beautifully. It looks like she is starting puberty. I guess she is probably already very popular with the boys.

Sarah gives me a big hug and exclaims, "Dr. Chris! It's so good to see you! Michael is in bed again with belly pain."

Rachel walks into the room to greet me. She looks worried and tired. Her shoulder length red hair is unkempt. A black apron is covering her black pants and yellow top. She is apparently in the middle of cooking dinner. "Welcome to our home! Thank you for stopping over!"

After some quick small talk about my trip, she gets to what is really on her mind, "I don't know what's wrong with Michael. As I told you over the phone, he's been sick a lot in the last three weeks."

As Rachel, followed by Sarah, takes me into the room I'll be sleeping in, she tells me more about Michael. "Last week, I took him to the hospital, thinking it was appendicitis. They did a blood test and an ultrasound, and both were normal. I haven't changed anything in his diet. I don't understand what's happening. Just to try something different, I put him on a gluten-free and a lactose-free diet, but it doesn't help. He still has this terrible belly pain."

We head to Michael's room, and Rachel calls out, "Michael, honey, Dr. Chris is here. Can she come and say hello?"

I hear a faint "Yes, Mom," and the three of us enter Michael's bedroom.

The bedroom walls are decorated with pictures of planes and helicopters. It makes me feel good that Michael has a special interest in his life. A dark-haired, eight year old boy with trendy-cut short brown hair is in bed, playing on an iPad what seems to be a loud, violent video game. I can hear lots of explosions, gunfire, and shouting. As Michael turns in my direction, I notice his clear brown eyes have an expression I have never seen in him before. I was hoping to see him happy, but instead, all I can see is darkness. Something bad is going on.

As I greet Michael and ask him how he is feeling, Sarah jumps in and, in a serious tone, suggests, "Maybe he should give his belly a voice!"

I smile. I have known Sarah and Michael since they were toddlers. They have gotten used to my unconventional healing secrets. And they know that I prescribe as little medication as possible. They have gotten used to giving various parts of their bodies a voice when they come to see me with ailments, and they have come to love it. It has allowed them to get to know their bodies better.

I love teaching kids how to handle symptoms of illness. The first ten years of a child's life determines a lot of what will happen during the rest of his life. It is in those first ten years that he can learn how to eat well, exercise well, and understand the way his body functions—or not. Those years also determine what he will teach his kids and grandkids. Because it is so important for their future, I don't mind investing a lot of my time in educating kids on how to eat healthily and handle symptoms the right way.

I love the fact that Sarah is suggesting that Michael give his body a voice. I want to compliment her. "That's a good idea Sarah, thank you!" I turn toward Michael and, with a smile, say, "Michael, as Dr. Sarah suggested, if your belly could talk, what would it say?"

Michael answers with a dull voice, not taking his eyes off his video game. "I don't know." That's all he will say, and he continues to shoot at whatever is on his iPad screen.

I am surprised that his belly doesn't know. This is so unlike Michael. In the past, he would always come up with some kind of explanation from his body. His dull voice is also surprising since he usually has a high-pitched voice coupled with a very bubbly attitude and a lot of energy and imagination. Whatever he is suffering from is serious. I am curious to examine him.

After asking him for permission to examine him, I grab his iPad, place it on his night stand, lift his t-shirt up, and expose his belly. I can see right away that it isn't distended. I warm my hands by rubbing them together, then I very gently place my right hand flat on his belly without any pressure and my left hand on top of my right hand. Michael reacts immediately with "Ouch!" It's a strange reaction because his belly isn't distended, and I haven't put any pressure on it yet. I did nothing that would make it hurt.

To measure his liver, I place my right hand on his right lower chest, fingers open, then, putting my right middle finger in between two ribs, I tap on it with my left middle finger going lower and lower at each tapping. The hollow sound of lungs suddenly gives way to dull, full sound. I have found the upper part of his liver. To feel its lower part, I place my right hand flat on his belly, press lightly and ask him to breathe deeply. Despite his "Ouch!" I find the lower part of his liver. It isn't enlarged. A good sign.

I move my fingers to the middle upper part of his belly, pressing very slightly again, checking his stomach. There too, he grimaces and gives out another "Ouch!" I move my fingers to the left upper quadrant, checking his spleen and left upper part of his bowel. To my surprise, there too is pain.

As I continue lower, I examine his left lower quadrant to check for lower bowel and right lower quadrant to rule out appendicitis. Extremely light pressure on both of those elicits pain. I am puzzled! All quadrants of Michael's abdomen are painful to the slightest touch, but his belly isn't distended and I hear normal gurgling which means there is no bowel obstruction.

What could possibly be the diagnosis? Could it still be appendicitis? Or maybe colitis or gastritis?

I ask Rachel if there has been any fever, nausea, vomiting, constipation, or diarrhea, but her response is negative. The only thing, she says is that one day, the infirmary called her because Michael's nose was bleeding. She picked him up early that day and kept cotton balls up in his nose a few hours. It only happened once.

I reflect that nose bleeds in kids can always happen, and if it only happened once to Michael, it doesn't worry me. I have to find another way to fish for clues. I ask Michael's mother when the pain started and whether some event she can recall coincided with the beginning of the pain.

Attentive mother that she is, Rachel remembers exactly the day it all started. "His belly pain started three weeks ago when he came back from school. He said he had a potato salad for lunch that didn't taste fresh."

I am perplexed. Three weeks is a long time for a belly pain due to bad food. Usually viral or bacterial gastro-enteritis resolve within a few days—unless, I think—the only thing that could take longer is a liver infection. I turn to Michael to examine his eyes. They look clear. No yellow there, which rules out a possible hepatitis. The mystery is still intact, hidden from me in spite of my efforts.

I finish my examination by inspecting the back of his throat, pressing slightly on the sides of his neck looking for lymph nodes and listening to his lungs and heart. Everything seems normal.

As I put my stethoscope back in my bag, Sarah speaks up. "Michael hasn't been able to go to school the last three weeks. He is going to be really behind!"

Interesting! I wonder if the belly pain is related to school. In the past, I have had several young patients with similar belly pains, and very often they were related to a teacher the child didn't like or was afraid of. Just the thought of going back to school and facing that teacher brought on the child's belly spasms.

Is that Michael's problem? Is he worried about something at school? It's a good bet that he is, because one of the most common ways that anxiety influences the body is by causing abdominal pain like Michael's. The anxiety promotes "spastic colon" (painful contractions of the large intestine) in response to elevated stress hormones. Anxiety and depression have also been shown to heighten people's *awareness* of bowel discomfort.

I decide to ask him directly if there is a teacher at school that he doesn't like, but he tells me there isn't. I decide to use one of my indirect tools to bypass his conscious defenses. This time, unlike with Mark, I don't think a walk in nature will do much good. Instead, I ask him to make me a drawing.

"Michael, if your belly can't have a voice, maybe it can make a drawing for me if I give you a paper and crayons."

Michael answers that he doesn't feel like drawing and would rather just play his video game. I don't give up. Instead I borrow some of Sarah's coloring supplies, some sheets of drawing paper and colorful crayons, and leave them next to his bed. In a casual manner I tell him that if his belly changes its mind, I would love it if it could make a drawing for me.

Michael seems to ignore my words and is already back to his video game. I leave his room followed by Rachel and Sarah.

I remain puzzled by Michael's attitude. I have always known him to be very talkative, even too talkative, when he is sick. His silence is unusual, as is the fact that his whole abdomen is sensitive to the slightest touch without bloating, abnormal mass, or fever.

As Rachel, Sarah, and I (Michael wasn't hungry and didn't want to join us) dine on our roasted chicken and mashed potatoes, Rachel says, "On weekends, for some reason, he has less pain, but he still doesn't talk the way he used to."

We all go to bed early that night. I reflect on the fact that on weekends, the pain is less, a fact that fits the avoiding school theory. I am determined to find a way to solve this mystery.

In the morning, I go to Michael's room to see how he feels.

Michael still looks drawn and rather lifeless, but he replies, "Good!" Then to my surprise, he reaches under his bed, grabs the paper I gave him the night before and hands it to me and immediately turns away and starts playing on his iPad.

I glance at the sheet of paper. "Great! Your belly did a drawing . . ." I can't finish my sentence. I am stunned into silence. I can't utter a word as I stare at Michael's drawing.

I gave Michael plenty of colorful crayons, but he only used two colors: black and red. I see what seems to be a little person standing upright with a red cloud of drops falling on him surrounded by five large angry, strange-looking faces. As I look at Michael's drawing, to my surprise, he grabs it and turns it upside down. It now shows the same little person but this time hanging upside down with red drops falling on the ground and making a puddle with the five angry large faces surrounding him. The new perspective makes a big difference. "Is this the way I should look at your drawing?" I ask.

As he nods, I begin to examine the drawing more closely. The large faces have sharp teeth and arched eyebrows. Vampires? What does the red color represent? Could it be blood? That is certainly worrisome. Is Michael the little person in the middle being attacked, or is he one of the big faces attacking somebody smaller?

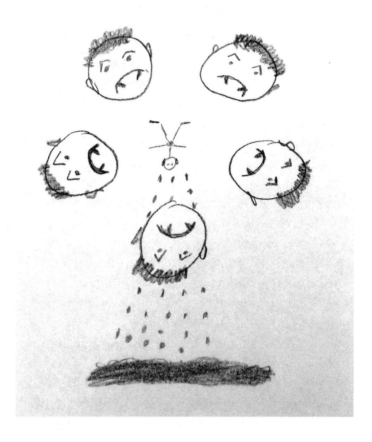

I look at Michael. He seems deep into his video game again. Despite being worried, I decide to play the cool-friend card and look at the video game with him. It is a war game, and he is relentlessly shooting down virtual enemies.

After a few minutes, I decide it is time to probe. The best way to know exactly what the drawing represents is to ask the little artist. In order for him to disclose as much as possible, I want to look excited about his drawing, so I ask in a forced, joyful voice, "I am so happy your belly did a drawing for me! Can you tell me what it represents?"

Michael is silent, concentrating on his video game. He is not showing any interest in commenting on his drawing.

I decide to change subject. "How is your belly pain this morning, Michael?"

Without lifting his head up to look at me, he replies, "Same."

I look at him attentively. From past experiences, I know that kids his age usually project themselves into the drawing. The implication is troubling.

Could the angry faces represent his family? When there is violence towards children, domestic abuse is often the cause. Is his family hurting him? An uneasy feeling grows in *my* stomach as I worry about the possibility of domestic violence. As a physician, I am a "mandated reporter," which means that, by law, I am compelled to report cases of child abuse.

But no. I have been close to Rachel for years, and I don't really believe that she, or Sarah for that matter, are capable of hurting him. Maybe Michael's dad's new family? I remember that his dad left Rachel three years ago. He had since remarried a younger woman with no children. But I don't remember Michael's dad as being a violent man. He left Rachel because he had fallen in love with his young secretary.

My thoughts turn to problems outside the home. Is he being threatened by multiple people, or is he one of the aggressors in the drawing? I consider this at length and finally decide that the most probable explanation is that Michael is the little person in the middle of the drawing. As I am about to probe Michael, Rachel and Sarah enter the room.

Rachel smiles and says, "Good morning. I am going to drop Sarah off at school. Can I leave you with Michael for half-an-hour? I'll be back in no time."

I am happy to be alone with Michael. The timing is perfect. I wait until I hear the door slammed shut. Then I begin my inquiry, taking a direct approach. "Michael, is that you, the little person hanging upside down in the middle of the drawing?"

Michael still shooting bad guys left and right silently nods his head. I know I am on to something. I need to probe deeper. "I am going to take a guess here, Michael. The people around you—are they threatening you?"

Still playing his video game, he nods his head. But my question has had an effect, and his focus on the game seems a bit less intense. A good sign. I continue, pointing at the angry faces on the drawing, "Are those boys bullying you in school?"

Michael continues to stare at the screen, pretending he is still playing his video game, but I can see he has stopped. I am probably zeroing in on the problem. He responds to my question with an affirmative nod.

I decide to go for broke. "Michael, are there boys bullying you every day at school and threatening to hurt you if you tell anybody? Is that the reason you're having belly pain and why you don't want to go to school anymore?"

Michael looks at me straight in the eye. I can see his fear, the same expression I saw the previous night. I described it then as darkness when in reality, it is deep and intense fear. He nods his head once more. He is beginning to whimper.

In order for him to open up to me, I need to reassure him that nothing bad will happen to him or his family if he confides in me, and maybe later tells his mom. I explain that bullies employ terrible threats to scare their victims. When they are exposed, and their parents and even the police get involved, they can do no more harm.

It is time to ask him to be the little person in the middle of his drawing, to give it a voice in the first person. After what seems like forever, Michael starts talking. "I am so little compared to them. I am so scared. I am hanging upside down, my nose is bleeding. I am afraid they are going to drop me on the ground. My head will hit the ground and explode." He is sobbing and shaking.

Yes, it all makes sense now. The drawing is of Michael being harmed, dropped head first, and his nose or his head is bleeding.

A puddle of blood is collecting at the bottom of the drawing. I am very touched by Michael's trust. I sit next to him on the bed and take him in my arms. It is important that I reassure him again.

He slowly relaxes. After a few moments of silence he has apparently decided he can trust me, and he describes how he is being bullied everyday by three older boys who have formed a gang with two others. They are very powerful and are also threatening other kids. He describes how they hurt him with "Indian rubs" on his ears (rubbing his ears fast and hard until they turn red) that hurt so much and leave no mark; with "noogies," hitting their knuckles on his chest, arms and legs; how he was "pantsied" (pulling his pants down) and hung by his feet upside down over a third story window, as they threatened to drop him. He also describes how they have repeatedly threatened to kill him and his family if he says anything against them.

I now understand the situation. He is afraid for his family as well as for himself. His only way out is to not go to school anymore. He has probably figured out that he can use his very real belly pain as an excuse to miss school. The unconscious could be causing a sustained release of stress hormones in order to keep the belly pain going—an unending reason to stay home. It's a well-known phenomenon in kids called secondary gains when they unconsciously sustain a "bad thing" (the belly ache) in order to bring about a "good thing" (staying home and out of harm's way).

I wonder now about the apparent puddle of blood in the drawing. Does it represent a nose bleed, or is his unconscious signaling something much worse, such as internal bleeding? I must find out.

After I ask Michael about the blood, he explains: One day, the boys took turns giving his ears Indian rubs. It hurt so much that he screamed and his nose started to bleed. To shut him up, the boys put paper in his mouth then hung him upside down, which made the nose bleed worse. As blood puddled on the ground, the boys became frightened, put him flat on his back and ran away. Michael thought that he was going to die. When he was able to pick himself up, he wisely went to the infirmary, and Rachel was called to come and get him. But he didn't tell anything to the school nurse or to Rachel.

With a trembling voice he asks, "Dr. Chris, are you sure that they won't kill my mom and Sarah?" I reassure him that they will be perfectly safe from these bullies.

And I myself am reassured that the blood in the drawing is only a nose bleed.

I let some time pass. Then I ask, "Can your belly now tell me what is going on with it? Belly, have you been hit by the bullies?"

Michael looks at me directly in the eyes. I now see the Michael I used to know, talkative and always having answers for me. Giving voice to his belly, he says, "Yes, they hit me, but only at the beginning. Now, I am in pain about going back to school. I don't want to go back. I hate school." I am relieved that I have heard nothing worse from Belly. I thank Michael and his belly for being so open and honest with me, and I ask his permission to tell his mom when she comes back.

When Rachel returns, I take her aside, show her Michael's drawing, and tell her the whole story. She is horrified and cries out, "I had no idea! Oh my God!" She runs to Michael's room and takes him in her arms.

Rachel is in tears now. "Is this true, Michael, what Dr. Chris is telling me?" Michael confirms the whole story.

The following day, after taking me to the airport, Rachel goes to see the principal of Michael's school.

When I call from Paris, a week later, Rachel tells me that the bullies have been expelled, but Michael is not going back. She has decided to home-school Michael as he remains terrified about returning to the school. The good news is that his belly pain has disappeared.

In Michael's case, we have seen how useful and effective art can be in helping to make a diagnosis.

My secret healing techniques, however, are not limited just to having patients draw or paint. I have used other kinds of artistic expression as well. It all depends on the patient.

If the patient likes to sing or play a musical instrument, asking him to create an improvised song can be as useful and helpful as a drawing. Not only can it help in making a diagnosis, but also can be used for treating the problem. Here, I am my own case study.

I remember when my late husband was fighting against cancer, and I was very depressed. In order to cope with the situation and avoid taking antidepressants, I had weeks where I would go to my car every morning, drive half an hour, create songs and lyrics in tune with my mood, and sing them at the top of my lungs. I did not censor myself; all words that rose spontaneously, no matter how weird, became my lyrics. The songs I created were beautiful to my ears even though I know nothing about music, and even though, if someone had overheard me, they probably would not like what they heard. But my improvisational singing was very therapeutic.

Some people like to dance, and dancing can be as effective as drawing or music. For patients who love to trip the light fantastic, I ask them to dance out their emotions. The act is both diagnostic and therapeutic because spontaneous movement can provide a direct link to the unconscious and become a healthy expression of repressed feelings.

## Healing-Secret Exercises

*Here is a practical exercise in drawing to discover hidden parts of yourself:*

Take a piece of paper, gather a few colorful crayons, and draw whatever comes to mind.

When you are finished drawing, focus on one object you have drawn that calls for your attention. Give that object a voice in the first person.

For example, if you draw a rabbit, say, "I am a rabbit. . . ."
Or if you draw a sun, say, "I am a sun. . . ." Then describe
yourself in relation to the surroundings you created in
your drawing. Continue by saying "I am feeling. . . . or I
wish. . . ."

By opening this door to your unconscious, you might
discover parts of yourself that were deeply buried inside.
The journey into yourself can be fascinating.

If you are sick or in pain, it might open doors you didn't
know existed and help you find solutions you hadn't
thought about.

*Here's another practical exercise to learn about something deep inside:*

If you feel more like singing or playing an instrument,
create a song from scratch. Invent the music and the lyrics.
Don't think too much.

Sing or play whatever comes to mind. Let your music
match exactly what your body is experiencing. Whatever
you create will be beautiful because it will come from deep
inside of you. This is how the most successful songs came
to life.

You'll find your music-making to be extremely therapeutic.

If you prefer dancing, then dance your emotion, dance
your symptom. (If you are in pain, perform a very slow
dance.) Then give words to your dance.

By giving your pain an outlet, its intensity will decrease. By
creating words for a song or a dance, you might find the
core origin of your medical problem and the best way to
cure it.

# 9

# A Dialogue with Death

AT THE END of October each year Mexicans put on macabre death masks and march in parades as skeletons. They prepare gifts for departed loved ones, visit cemeteries, and spend time with the dead.

This unusual festival called Dias los Muertos should be thought of not as a preoccupation with death, but rather as a way to embrace *living*. Curator Encarnacion Teruel of the Mexican Fine Arts Center Museum in Chicago explains the holiday this way:

> "It gives you an opportunity to feel good about someone's life, beyond mourning. It gives you a chance to affirm life by recognizing death."

This point of view makes a lot of sense once we admit that nothing makes us appreciate what we have as much as losing it.

* We don't fully appreciate our job until we lose it and have to struggle to make ends meet.
* We don't fully appreciate a friend until she or he moves away.
* We don't fully appreciate our youth until we are old.

But how does this work with regard to our own life, our very existence? Life is not something we can "lose" and then, after death, look back and appreciate it and miss it.

So we will never have the same opportunity to fully appreciate life the same way we get to appreciate things like a lost job or lost friends.

The Mexican festival recognizes this. And the last secret I have to share with you does too.

For patients going through especially frightening medical ordeals, I have discovered that focusing attention on death can promote both healing and quality of life.

I have saved this discussion for the end of the book for a reason. All of the secrets I have shared so far, in one way or another, are about getting patients to shift their point of view by becoming the voice of their body, or, the voice of others. In doing this, they can get past emotional defenses and other obstacles that obscure the truth about their health, their bodies, their emotional lives from them.

So, while we can't just leave or lose our life (that's called death!) in order for us to appreciate it, there is a way we can shift our way of looking at and thinking about life. We can do this by seeing our life from death's point of view!

But how is it possible to do that?

I have found a way to create a situation that allows us to understand better the loss of life and the end of our own life—and it is by having a conversation with death.

If we could talk to death itself, if we could have a conversation with the force that will someday take us away from everyone and everything we love, surprisingly enough, we might discover some unexpected positive insights.

In this chapter, I explore the idea of conversing with death in my case of Susan. Under my guidance she met with the personification of death, spoke with it, and came away with a new point of view that changed her life for the better.

## Susan's Story

Susan was seventy-six years old when she noticed a little bit of red color in her stools. She thought she had eaten too many cherries and laughed about it. One month later, she got up in the morning, and after using the bathroom saw that the water in the toilet bowl was pink. Cherry season was long over. Was it blood? She started shivering! No, it couldn't possibly be blood! What if it was? She shook her head, tried to forget about the incident and went shopping.

A retired math teacher, she had been married for five years in the early 1980s and had two daughters. At that time her daughter, Emma, forty-two, was married with a ten-year-old son, and the other daughter, Laura, was forty and unmarried. After her second daughter was born, Susan and her husband grew apart. They eventually divorced, and her life has since been uncomplicated and centered on raising her two daughters and working at the local high school until her retirement at age sixty-three.

Her biggest pleasure was playing bridge with her friends. She found that her math background was a tremendous asset for the game.

That day she went shopping, she purchased a new pair of black high heeled dressy shoes to go with the new blue dress she planned to wear at her grand-niece's upcoming wedding. When she got back home from shopping, she prepared a healthy dinner, read for a while, and went to bed.

The following morning, there it was again—what seemed to be blood in her stools. She had tried to forget about it, forcing herself to believe it was just a bad dream that would soon go away. But it didn't. She realized that she had to face reality and made an appointment with her primary care physician.

At the appointment a week later, the doctor examined her and suggested that she was probably suffering from hemorrhoids. But to be completely sure, he recommended a colonoscopy. She'd never had one before, even though she knew that after the age fifty, regular colonoscopies are recommended. She refused to expose herself to the aggravating preparation of a day devoted to drinking a vile liquid that aids in emptying the bowels.

Once again Susan decided to hold off having the colonoscopy, convincing herself that the blood was merely her hemorrhoids acting up. She began applying a new antihemorrhoid ointment, and was relieved that the bleeding seemed to decrease over the next few days.

Unfortunately, two months later the bleeding increased, and she began to feel abnormally tired. She became very frightened when she experienced shortness of breath after merely walking up a few stairs in her home.

Susan made another appointment with her primary care physician who sent her for a blood test. When the result came, it showed severe anemia. She had to go to the hospital immediately for an urgent blood transfusion.

Susan panicked. What if she had colon cancer? No, that couldn't possibly happen to her! She had never smoked, never drank alcohol, and almost always ate healthy food!

After receiving the blood transfusion, and at the urging of her doctor, she finally agreed to have a colonoscopy the following day. The preparation was not as bad as she expected, and she didn't feel any pain during the procedure.

The results were not encouraging. Her gastroenterologist told her that he found a large ulcerated mass in her lower sigmoid colon that looked like cancer. He was waiting for the biopsy results, but said there was no time to lose and referred her to a colorectal surgeon.

That evening, the surgeon visited her in her hospital room to tell her that she would probably need to have the tumor removed as well as a large part of her bowel around the tumor. He scheduled her for surgery in two weeks.

When pathology results came back, they showed, as expected, an aggressive colon cancer. More work-up was done, and fortunately abdominal scans showed that the disease had not spread. But since her cancer was so aggressive, she was told she would need chemotherapy and radiation therapy after the surgery.

Susan became extremely upset. She became distraught and began agitating herself with disturbing thoughts: What if this was going to be the end of her life? What if death was around the corner? She had never thought about her own death. Yes, she had seen her mother and father die, but to her those were normal, expected events of old age. Her own dying, she believed, would be neither normal nor expected at this time. It was way too soon!

Susan became so anxious that she couldn't sleep at night. When she got up in the morning, she was already exhausted. She could not imagine how she was going to deal with her situation. She was paralyzed with fear and felt herself falling apart, losing hope, losing her health, losing her sanity. It all became unbearable.

That's when she came to my office, which was decorated that day with pink roses brought in by a grateful patient.

At noon on a Friday, the week before Easter, my receptionist opens my door to let in a tall slim woman in her seventies, wearing a long black coat. As she removes the coat and places it on the back of her chair before sitting across from my desk, I look at her. Her short, curly dark brown hair suits her. Her lips have bright red lipstick, and her brown eyes are circled with black eyeliner, which would look very nice if in addition they were not also circled with deep purplish lines. The purplish lines make her look tired. The dull brown shirt she wears on top of black pants accentuate her unfortunate appearance.

Susan explains that she is scheduled for surgery the following week. She will begin chemotherapy and radiation therapy a month after the surgery.

I ask her why she has made this appointment with me, and she replies that her pharmacist, located in the building next to my office, referred her to me when she asked for an over-the-counter antianxiety drug. The pharmacy knows me well since I send my patients there for prescription medicine as well as over-the-counter homeopathic remedies. The pharmacist has heard through my other patients about my unconventional methods for dealing with anxiety, especially with anxiety about death.

Susan explains that she believes she is facing death. When she goes to bed at night, she is scared she won't wake up, so part of her doesn't want to fall asleep. During the day, she is exhausted. Thinking that she might die from her cancer, from her surgery, or from her chemo frightens her to no end.

As a physician, my duty is to help patients prevent their dying, and I have worked diligently at that all my life. But I have found that avoiding the very subject of their passing is a mistake for patients who face the real possibility of imminent death. Doctors generally wish to avoid the subject. But sometimes avoiding death is not the answer; confronting death is what is necessary.

So I prefer to guide my terminal patients to use death to their own advantage, to find the ways in which the very idea of death can illuminate and strengthen the rest of their lives.

Susan believes she is "facing death." Her fear is justified since her body knows she could die from her cancer or from complications of surgery or chemotherapy. In such cases, I have great results from having the patient talk to death directly. Since dealing with death is part of being alive, and sooner or later, everybody will have to face it, I have the patient imagine that death is a friendly entity.

I begin by asking Susan, "I understand you are facing death. Can you imagine literally and physically facing death? What color would death be? Maybe dark grey?" As I say this, I grab a dark grey pillow from my pillow closet and place it on a chair that I bring in front of where she is sitting.

This is practical visualization, and I use it because it turns a theoretical idea into something that a patient can see and even touch. Practical visualization changes all dynamics. As for color, I choose grey for death, a somewhat more friendly color than black, and an important consideration since I am planning to have Susan befriend it. I continue, "If you could talk to death as if it were an acquaintance what would you say?"

Susan looks at me with panic in her eyes as I bring the dark grey pillow chair in front of her. She gazes on the dark pillow, and I see her body stiffen. She sits up straight, clenches her hands on her lap, crosses her ankles under her chair, and opens her eyes wide. She remains silent and takes a few deep breaths.

I decide to remain silent too, giving her time to get used to the idea of facing death and waiting until she relaxes a bit.

After a few very long seconds, I see her back is loosening up a bit, and her breathing is returning to normal. I want her to relax even more, so I say in a soft, gentle voice, "Death is nothing personal, Susan. Death is part of everyone's life."

Susan continues staring at the dark pillow a few more long seconds, and then she says, "Doc, there are two parts of me, one that wants to run away with fear and the other that wants to get closer to the dark pillow and maybe even touch it. It's a very strange feeling."

Sometimes when something we fear in theory comes close to us and becomes more real, our reaction can be surprising and unexpected. In Susan's case, it is surprising that one part of her wants to get closer and even touch the dark pillow. This reaction could be important for her treatment. Yet, since she has expressed the reactions of two different parts of her, my goal is to give both of those parts a voice, to consider them as two distinct entities.

For maximum visual impact, I bring another chair and place it next to her. "Here is the other you," I say. "Let's make it the you that wants to run away with fear. Let's give it a voice."

The reason I want her to start with her fearful entity is to get it out of the way so that the other entity, the least well-known one, the one I am most interested in, will be free to speak.

Susan sits on the new chair (I'll call it the "fear chair") facing the dark pillow and begins, "I am scared of you. I really don't want to have anything to do with you. I hate you. You took my mom, then my dad, then my best friend! How could you do this to me?" Susan's face is beginning to turn red and tears are starting to fall. She suddenly gets up. "I am running away from you," she cries, and walks toward the door.

While she is standing near the exit door, I ask her about what happened to her best friend, and she explains that she died six months ago from ovarian cancer. My heart goes out to her as I express my condolences. I thank her for her willingness to become the voice of her fear and ask if there is anything more this part of her wants to say. When she shakes her head in silence, I ask her to come back and sit on the chair next to the fear chair and explore what that unexpected, surprising, separate entity of her wants to say.

She slowly walks back and sits on the other chair (I'll call it the "gutsy Susan" chair). "It is so strange," she says as she faces the dark pillow again. "This part of me almost wants to touch the dark pillow." She extends her right hand towards the dark pillow to the point of almost touching it, then withdraws quickly. "No, I don't want to touch it!" She looks at me as if to ask, "What should I do now?"

She is still sitting on the "gutsy Susan" chair facing the dark grey pillow. Now I want her to turn this encounter with death into a positive one. "If you had something to gain and to learn from talking to death, what do you think it would it be?"

Susan remains silent, looking at the dark grey pillow and taking a few deep breaths. I remain silent too, focusing on her body language. Her back is straight, and she moves her hands that were resting on her lap up in front of her eyes, perhaps a signal from her unconscious that it really doesn't want to proceed. Her legs and feet still rest gently on the floor.

Susan seems deeply absorbed in her thoughts. Then, moving her hands away from her eyes, she places them in front of her chest in a prayer position. Looking at the dark grey pillow, she says, "I know I am going to be taken by you one day. I know death is inevitable. I just wish it won't be soon. I wish I can have surgery, finish chemo, and have time to enjoy life before you take me."

The prayer position in which she has unconsciously placed her hands is very meaningful. I interpret it as her begging death to give her more time—a bit of body language that matches her words. It tells me that her unconscious and consciousness are in unison.

Now I must ask her to switch places again and sit right on the dark grey pillow, the "death pillow." I want her to take on death's point of view and respond to Susan's supplication. People are always taken aback when I ask them to take on the role of death, but it is a move that makes the treatment more effective.

Susan is understandably perplexed, and we discuss the idea for a few more minutes. I try to reassure her and apparently succeed as she gets up, though reluctantly, and places herself gingerly on the dark grey pillow.

I notice her demeanor changes as soon as she changes seats. Her body is more rigid, her back stiffer, and her eyes look colder. After a few seconds, she starts speaking, and her voice is deeper. Looking at the "gutsy Susan" chair she says, "Susan, I am for sure going to take you one day, but your time hasn't come yet. Now is the time for you to appreciate being alive. But you take everything for granted and don't understand how good your life is. Maybe now, before your surgery, you can start enjoying being alive. Maybe you can begin to appreciate the simple pleasures of life like going for a walk on a warm spring afternoon, or just spending time with family."

Sitting on the "death pillow" and taking death's point of view creates a leap into the unknown, and often produces spectacular results. Imagine! Death is criticizing Susan for not taking time to appreciate life! Who would have thought? The sentiment is wonderful and may well lead the way to a better future for Susan.

Once Susan is done speaking from death's point of view, I ask her to switch back to the "gutsy Susan" chair. She is still deep in her thoughts, but she gets up and does what I ask anyway.

After a few moments of silence, she speaks to the dark grey pillow, to death. "So, I just need to accept you, and maybe if I look at my future with you next to me, it will feel different."

This is a profound insight, and I want to reinforce it. Knowing how it is important to visualize everything, I pick up death's chair with the dark grey pillow and bring it next to Susan. This is an important move suggested by her, and I want to take advantage of what this different point of view may offer. I am trying to represent the idea that now death is not in front of her, calling for a confrontation, it is besides her, as an ally would be.

With this new configuration in place, I stay silent, waiting. After taking a few deep breaths, Susan takes in the new situation, with death no longer threatening her. She says, "This changes everything." She begins to focus on the pink roses in a purple vase on a table against the near wall. "Those roses are so beautiful." She suddenly gets up, walks toward the roses, grabs the vase, brings it back with her, and sits on the "gutsy Susan" chair again next to the dark grey pillow. She places the vase on her lap. "For some reason, sitting next to this dark pillow makes those roses look more gorgeous." She puts her nose up to them. "And they smell so good." Then without thinking, she places her hand on the dark grey pillow next to her.

That is a great unconscious move. As soon as she realizes she is touching the "death pillow," she quickly takes her hand off. I have to smile.

She seems much less frightened now, and that is what I hoped would happen. I have found that the thing we fear most can have a positive side, and provide unexpected benefits, but we need to work to find them. In Susan's case, accepting the inevitability of

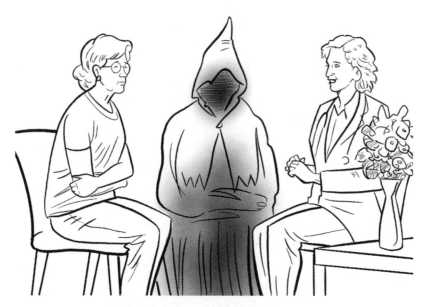

*"I see you are afraid of dying, but if you could have
a conversation with death,
how do you imagine it would go?"*

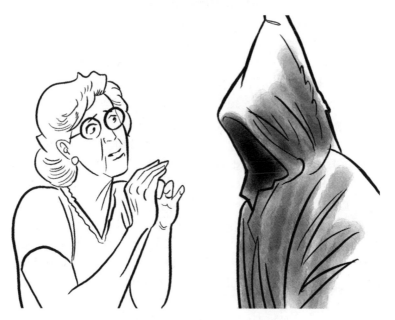

*"I am so scared of you! There are so many things
I would like to do before you take me!"*

death is helping her to see all that is good in life. This is the result I am looking for, and Susan confirms that we have arrived there.

She says, "I think that with the dark pillow next to me, I can appreciate life more intensely, knowing that it could be taken away from me at any moment."

Yes, this is it. All too often, people don't recognize the wonder of life and all gifts life brings them. They take life for granted, not understanding that it can be taken from them or their loved ones at any moment. Only when they do understand these possibilities can they start appreciating every single pleasure in life. This is one of the insights provided by celebrating the Dias Los Muertos rituals I described at the beginning of the chapter.

I ask Susan, "If you can concentrate on the joy of still being alive, what would be most pleasurable for you?"

Susan takes a few deep breaths. Smiling as she looks at the dark grey pillow next to her, she says, "Death is right. I have never really appreciated being alive before. I want to spend more time with my daughters and with my grandson. I want to have a big party and invite all my friends and family to celebrate my life."

"If I die—when I die—all my friends will get together at my funeral, but it won't be too much fun for me! I really should have a party while I'm still alive so I can enjoy it too." She laughs. "There are other things I want to do. I want to go on a cruise to Alaska and take my daughters with me. I have always dreamed of lots of travel. There are so many places I want to see. I keep putting it off, but no more. I promise myself that if I survive this cancer, I'll book a cruise to Alaska."

Her tone of voice is now cheerful, and her eyes are sparkling, a beautiful sight. She seems suddenly to have been energized. I am so pleased. My unconventional approach has turned her paralyzing feeling of fear of death into a positive feeling of the joy of being alive.

She continues. "I am ready to fight! I am ready for surgery and chemo! I will be strong, and I will beat this because I want to do so much with my life."

Her voice is not only cheerful. it is strong and has the tone of a winner. My own heart is full of joy since I feel I have accomplished my mission. "Well, Susan, you are going to have a lot of time to appreciate life. In the time before your surgery, then between surgery and chemo, then during chemo, then after all treatments are done, I recommend you focus on every simple and small pleasure of life."

She nods with a smile. "I can do that!"

When Susan leaves my office, she looks radiant. She seems to be glowing with hope.

That same evening, when I am home, I remember my own dealings with death.

For a long time after my previous husband passed away from brain cancer at the age of fifty-six, I thought I was sharing my bed with death. Not only was I devastated because I had lost the love of my life, I was also afraid I was going to die shortly after him even though I was not sick. It was an unreasonable and uncontrollable fear.

I started having frequent sore throats and bronchitis. The fear and the illnesses continued until one day I decided that, instead of being scared of death, I would try befriending it.

After taking myself through a session similar to Susan's, with death by my side, I gained a very different vision of my life. Death became my friend, reminding me never to take anything for granted. Each morning I woke up happy and thankful that I was given one more day on earth. I started appreciating fully every single minute of my life, making each second count, making each second special. I took long lingering walks along the ocean, taking time to touch the sand, listen to the waves and the seagulls, taste and smell the salty air, feel the warmth of the sun on my

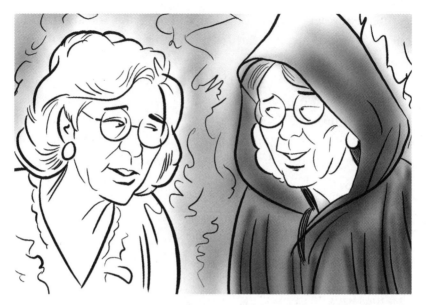

*Death replies: "Well, you have had many opportunities to do those things, but you have never done them, and you have never enjoyed your life fully! Can this change?"*

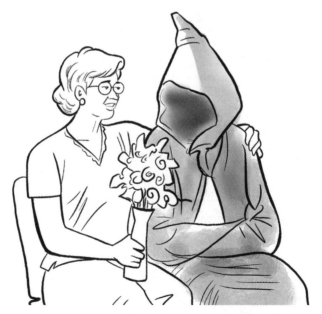

*Yes, this can change! With you by my side to remind me how precious life is, I will now live my life fully and appreciate every single minute of it!"*

skin. I cooked exquisite meals for myself every night. I took my good china out of the closet and ate from beautiful plates with real silver forks, spoons and knives, drank in crystal glasses, burned artistically decorated candles, and put in vases sumptuous fresh roses from my garden.

I lived as if each dinner was my last dinner, as if each walk was my last walk. I talked to all my friends and thanked them for their friendship. Neither past nor future existed anymore. I was totally in the present moment and enjoying it tremendously.

Little by little, I felt my emotional and physical strength increase every day. Eventually, my approach to life and death brought me back to balance and to health.

The change affected my medical practice. I took more time seeing each patient, focusing on his or her needs. Bringing my patients back to health gave me intense inner satisfaction, emotional strength, and even better health.

Ultimately, befriending death made me stronger than I ever was before.

As for Susan, several months after our last appointment, I received a postcard from Alaska where she was enjoying her long wished for cruise with her daughters.

Susan had her surgery, then her chemo and radiation therapy. The treatments worked, and she is now cancer free, enjoying every single minute of her life. She didn't just survive. Because of her life-affirming encounter with death, she also positively thrives! Now she even goes around to everyone who will listen to her to urge them to get a colonoscopy on a regular basis after the age of fifty.

Although I will never know for certain what role Susan's emotional acceptance of death played on her health, it is likely that her acceptance boosted her immune system by lessening negative pressure on the system from the chronic stress of worrying about death.

When people feel helpless and uncertain, elevated stress hormones depress their immune system, making them even more vulnerable to cancer and infection. This is a double whammy for cancer patients because they depend heavily on their immune system both to fight off their disease and to combat infections that are common with chemotherapy.

Conversely, when people feel they are empowered rather than helpless, their level of stress decreases.

By actively taking on death, rather than helplessly fearing it, Susan shifted from helplessness to empowerment. And, by taking her life into her own hands, and committing to enjoy it to its fullest, she gained more certainty about what her future held for her. Both of these shifts in point of view lessened her stress and, potentially, boosted her immune function.

Sometimes cancer wins no matter what positive emotional adjustments a patient makes, so patients should never blame themselves when treatments fail. But recent medical research suggests that cancer patients with lower levels of stress have lower death rates after treatments like chemotherapy. And, certainly, the quality of life of cancer patients who lower their stress is better than for those who struggle with stress.

Aware of this, I always work to reduce the stress of patients who are facing life-threatening illnesses and the debilitating therapies that are used to treat them.

Sometimes those patients are not as open to having direct conversations with death as Susan. I cannot blame them. After all, the prospect of death is incredibly frightening, and some people just want to hide from it.

With such patients, I get good results by asking them to project themselves into the future, coaxing them to imagine they are ninety-nine years old and on their death bed. I choose a pillow of a different color for their elderly, near-death self and ask them to create a dialogue between the person they are now and that very old projected wise and know-it-all senior. I ask them, "What advice can your ninety-nine-year-old self give your present self?"

This method produces a shift in perception in my patients. They look at the problem in a new and different way, and often priceless, ingenious solutions result.

With other patients whose symptoms started when they were children, I ask them to project themselves into the past instead of the future and encourage them to imagine they can talk to their young self at whatever age their symptoms began. A dialogue between their child self and their present self provides that valuable shift in temporal perception of the issues causing their illness and often uncovers innovative solutions.

I want to conclude this chapter, and this book, by emphasizing a belief that I hold strongly. It is a belief that runs throughout all of my work on healing the body and my focus on uncovering the emotional underpinnings of physical suffering:

*You have as much—or more—power over your illness than any doctor.*

In the face of disease, you can transform yourself from helplessness to empowerment, from uncertainty to certainty, and from hopelessness to hopefulness by shifting your point of view away from your mind, with all of its defenses, denials, and cluelessness about your body. You can make this shift of perspective by becoming a part of your body that confronts your mind, by becoming multiple parts of your body that confront your multiple "selves," by becoming part of your dreams or a part of nature or drawings that you make. You can even do this, as I have just shown, by becoming death or projecting yourself into the future or the past.

But however you choose do it, do it to regain your health!!

My healing secrets are now *your* healing secrets. Use them to live a happier, healthier life!

## A Healing-Secret Exercise

*Here's a practical exercise for changing perspectives about death:*

Project yourself in the future and imagine you are ninety-nine-years-old on your death bed.

Choose a pillow of the color of your choice for your ninety-nine year old self and place it in front of you.

Talk to that pillow. What can you tell your ninety-nine-years-old?

When you are done talking to your ninety-nine-year-old, switch pillows and sit on your wise, know-it-all, ninety-nine-year-old pillow. Take a few deep breaths to allow yourself to be in character.

If your ninety-nine-year-old self could converse with your present self, what advice would it give you?

Be free to use talking, screaming, crying, laughing as they spontaneously come to you.

Write down and use the advice you get from your ninety-nine-year-old wisely.

Even if you don't get any advice, just the fact of imagining yourself even just for a moment being 99 years old on a death bed and then being able to rewind and be yourself again will make you appreciate the present moment.

Life is short! Enjoy it to the max!

# ACKNOWLEDGMENTS

THE AUTHORS WISH to thank Kenzi Sugihara, Nancy Sugihara, and Kenichi Sugihara for believing enough in this book to publish it, Dave Conti for his wonderful editing, Jane Wesman for publicity, Jonathan Kirsch for providing legal counsel, Stephane Cojot-Goldberg for his photography, and Stanley Miller for his drawings. Dr. Gilbert also wishes to thank the thousands of patients she treated over the years who made her a better physician.

# SOURCES

## CHAPTER 1: SCREAM, CRY, AND LAUGH YOUR WAY TO HEALTH

3   **It's been estimated that around eighty percent:** Cummings, N.A. and VandenBos, G.R., "The Twenty Years Kaiser-Permanente Experience with Psychotherapy and Medical Utilization: Implications for National Health Policy and National Health Insurance." Health Policy Q. 1981 (2):159–175.

http://www.drweil.com/drw/u/ART00694/Stress.html.

9   **It turns out that when we think of things:** Locke, J., and Fehr, F., "Subvocalization of Heard or Seen Words Prior to Spoken or Written Recall," *The American Journal of Psychology*, 8(1) 1972, 63-68.

Aarons, L., "Subvocalization: Aural and Emg Feedback in Reading," first published in 1971 *Perceptual and Motor Skills*, 33(1), 271-306.

9   **And, as in all cases of voluntary movement: Sarah Hawkins, "**Anatomy and Physiology of Human Respiration and Phonation," *Foundations of Speech Communication.* www.ling.cam.ac.uk/li9/m2_0809_ respirationandphonation_web.ppt.

10   **First, recent brain imaging research:** Lieberman, M. http://www.scn. ucla.edu/pdf/Kircanski(inpress)PsychSci.pdf.

http://www.science20.com/news/writing_down_feelings_really_does_ make_us_feel_better_study_says.

## CHAPTER 2: THE HEALING SECRETS THAT CHANGED MY LIFE

20   **In a typical example of Gestalt therapy:** Nevis, E., Introduction, in *Gestalt Therapy: Perspectives and Applications* Edwin Nevis (ed.). (Cambridge, MA: Gestalt Press, 2000) p. 3.

Mackewn, J., 1997 *Developing Gestalt Counseling* (London, UK: Sage publications; Bowman, C. Brownell, P., "Prelude to Contemporary Gestalt Therapy," Gestalt!, vol. 4, no. 3, 2000. available at http://www.g-gej.org/4-3/prelude.html.

23   **Were the kind of volatile emotions . . .** Tamar Pincus, A. Kim Burton, Steve Vogel, Andy P. Field, "A Systematic Review of Psychological Factors as Predictors of Chronicity/Disability in Prospective Cohorts of Low Back Pain," PSPINE Volume 27, Number 5, pp E109–E120.

Sarno, J., *Healing Back Pain: The Mind-Body Connection*, Mass Market Paperback, February 1, 2010.

27   **Some medical research suggests that emotional distress:** Sarno, J., *Healing Back Pain: The Mind-Body Connection*, February 1, 2010. Tamar Pincus, A. Kim Burton, Steve Vogel, Andy P. Field, "A Systematic Review of Psychological Factors as Predictors of Chronicity/Disability in Prospective Cohorts of Low Back Pain," SPINE Volume 27, Number 5, 2002, pp. E109–E120.

27   **When stress hormones such as adrenaline are released:** C. D. Marsden and J. C. Meadows, "The Effect of Adrenaline on the Contraction of Human Muscle," *Journal of Physiology.* Apr; 207(2), 1970: 429–448.

27   **Other studies have shown that hormones:** Katherine A. Gordon, Elizabeth Lebrun, and Marjana T., "Stress-Induced Hormones Cortisol and Epinephrine Impair Wound Epithelization Olivera Stojadinovic," *Advanced Wound Care*, New Rochelle, Feb; 1(1) (2012): 29–35.

https://www.researchgate.net/profile/George_Chrousos/publication/222358164_Stress_Hormones_Th1Th2_patterns_ProAntiinflammatory_Cytokines_and_Susceptibility_toDisease/links/00b7d520a3d50d85e0000000.pdf.

33   **In the USA alone, 1.3 million people:** Kohn, L.T., Corrigan, J.M., Donaldson, M.S., editors. *To Err is Human: Building a Safer Health System.* (National Academies Press (US), 2000.

33   **And 400,000 people per year die:** http://www.thenationaltriallawyers.org/2015/01/hospital-deaths/.

33   **Did you know that medical mistakes:** http://www.hospitalsafetyscore.org/newsroom/display/hospitalerrors-thirdleading-causeofdeathinus-improvementstooslow.

## CHAPTER 3: CONNECTING WITH OUR GUT FEELINGS

41    **This is it! This is the core of the problem!:** John C. Markowitz, and Barbara L. Milrod, "The Importance of Responding to Negative Affect in Psychotherapies," *American Journal of Psychiatry.* 168(2) (Feb., 2011): 124–128.

Joseph LeDoux, *The Emotional Brain: The Mysterious Underpinnings of Emotional Life* (Simon & Schuster, 2015).

42    **I remember that research done at Harvard University:** Masheb, R.M. & Grilo, C.M. "Emotional Overeating And Its Associations with Eating Disorder Psychopathology Among Overweight Patients With Binge Eating Disorder," *International Journal of Eating Disorders,* 39 (2006): 141-146. http://www.health.harvard.edu/newsletter_article/why-stress-causes-people-to-overeat.

44    **Dr. Stephen Rollnick and colleagues:** http://www.southbristolgptrainers.co.uk/Workshop%20200910/Documents%202010/BehChange.pdf.

45    **Studies show that our tone of voice . . .** Alex Pentland, (MIT Press, 2010). http://www.personal.reading.ac.uk/~sxs07itj/web/Educational_files/PYMONS_Lecture3_slides. pdf.

52    **Our metabolic rate steadily decreases with age:** Roberts, S.B., Rosenberg, I., "Nutrition and Aging: Changes in the Regulation of Energy Metabolism with Aging." Physiol Rev. 86(2) (April 2006): 651-67.

52    **In studies on monkeys:** http://www.nature.com/ncomms/2014/140401/ncomms4557/full/ncomms4557.html.

52    **The same results have been:** Heilbron, L, Revisson, E American, "Calorie Caloric Restriction and Aging: Review of the Literature and Implications for Studies in Humans," vol. 78 no. 3 (2003):361-369.

63    **And experiments have shown:** Meena Shah, Jennifer Copeland, Lyn Dart, Beverley Adams-Huet, Ashlei James, Debbie Rhea, "Slower Eating Speed Lowers Energy Intake in Normal-Weight But Not Overweight/Obese Subjects, March 2014 *Journal of the Academy of Nutrition and Dietetics,* Volume 114, Issue 3 (March 2014): 393-402.

## CHAPTER 4: SEX TALK

65    **Orgasms also inhibit activity in the "fear center":** http://ejop.psychopen.eu/article/view/430/html.

66    **For these reasons, satisfying sex:** Brody, S. Biological Psychology, March
      2000.

      Light, K. Biological Psychology, April 2005.

      Charnetski, C. Psychological Reports, June 2004.

      Ebrahim, S. *Journal of Epidemiology and Community Health,* February 2002.

      Mulhall, J. *Journal of Sexual Medicine,* online Feb. 8,  2008.

      Meston, C. Archives of Sexual Behavior, August 2007.

      Zak, P. PLoS One, online Nov. 7, 2007.

      Uryvaev, Y. Bulletin of Experimental Biology and Medicine, November
      1996.

      Leitzmann, M. Journal of the American Medical Association, April 7,
      2004.

      Giles, G. BJU International, August 2003.

      American Cancer Society: "Ways of Dealing with Specific Sexual
      Problems."

      Lancel, M. Regulatory Peptides, July 15, 2003.

66    **Research has found that women:** Hui Liu and Linda Waite, http://
      paa2014.princeton.edu/papers/140290.

66    **It is estimated that fifty percent of people . . .** Kaare Christensen,
      Gabriele Doblhammer,  Roland Rau,  James W Vaupel, *Ageing
      Populations: The Challenges Ahead,* Lancet. (2009 Oct 3); 374(9696):
      1196–1208.

67    **When we shift to "Not Me":** Yontef, G., and Simkin, J. (1993). "An
      Introduction to Gestalt Therapy," Behavior, online. Retrieved July 2,
      2002, from http://www.behavior.net/gestalt.htm.

71    **The Kinsey Institute estimates . . .** Kim Wallen, Elisabeth A. Lloyd,
      "Female Sexual Arousal: Genital Anatomy and Orgasm in Intercourse,"
      Horm Behav. 2011 May; 59(5): 780–792. Published online 2010 Dec
      30. doi: 10.1016/j.yhbeh.2010.12.004.

71    **"When one spouse is sexually dissatisfied":** http://divorcebusting.com/
      pr_sex-starved_marriage.htm.

74     **The clitoris is exquisitely sensitive:** Carroll, *Sexuality Now, Embracing Diversity* (Wadsworth Publishing, 2012), pp.110–111, 252.

75     **Experts believe the fewer than five percent:** Nolen-Hoeksema, Susan, (New York, NY: McGraw-Hill Education., 2014), p. 368.

## CHAPTER 5: INNER GROUP THERAPY

93     **This development forced Zimbardo to end:** http://www.prisonexp. org/.

95     **The 2015-2020 Dietary Guidelines for Americans:** http://health.gov/ dietaryguidelines/2015/guidelines/.

97     **Daniel Kahneman, the Nobel Prize winning economist:** Tversky, A., and Kahneman, D. "Judgement Under Uncertainty: Heuristics and Biases Science," 185 (4157) 1974: 1124–1131. doi:10.1126/science.185.4157.11 24. PMID 17835457.

99     **Like Robin, most of us are oriented:** http://www.rochester.edu/pr/ Review/V74N4/0402_brainscience.html.

99     **Dr. Leslie Greenburg of York University has conducted:** Clarke, K. M., & Greenburg, L. S. (1986). "Differential Effects of the Gestalt Two-Chair Intervention and Problem Solving in Resolving Decisional Conflict." *Journal of Counseling Psychology,* 33(1), 11–15.

       F. N. Watts (Ed.), "Clinical Research on Gestalt Methods," in, *New Developments in Clinical Psychology,* Vol. II (New York: Wiley and the British Psychological Society) pp.5-19.

       Greenburg, L. S., Rice, L. N. (1981). The specific effects of a Gestalt intervention. Psychotherapy: Theory, Research, and Practice, 18, 31–37.

       P. L. Wachtel & S. B. Messer (Eds.), "Humanistic Approaches to Psychotherapy," *Theories of Psychotherapy: Origins and Evolution* (Washington, DC: American Psychological Association). pp. 97–129.

105    **Here is a possible explanation:** Schneiderman, N.; Ironson, G.; Siegel, S. D. (2005). "Stress And Health: Psychological, Behavioral, and Biological Determinants." *Annual Review of Clinical Psychology* 1: 607–628.

       Herbert, T. B. and Cohen, S.. "Stress And Immunity In Humans: A Meta-Analytic Review," (1993).

Psychosomatic Medicine 55 (4) 364–379.

"Black PH Stress and The Inflammatory Response: A Review of Neurogenic Inflammation." *Brain Behav Immun.* 2002 Dec;16(6):622-53.

http://www.psychiatrictimes.com/psychotic-affective-disorders/ psychodermatology-when-mind-and-skin-interact#sthash.BduWI9mD. dpuf.

http://www.psychodermatology.net/pdfs/ESDaP_Zaragoza_Abstracts. pdf.

http://www.psychiatrictimes.com/psychotic-affective-disorders/ psychodermatology-when-mind-and-skin-interact.

108   **It offers hints about why Robin's Skin:** http://www.psychodermatology. net/pdfs/ESDaP_Zaragoza_Abstracts.pdf.

http://www.psychiatrictimes.com/psychotic-affective-disorders/ psychodermatology-when-mind-and-skin-interact.

108   **In psychiatry, problems such as Robin's:** Henry E. Adams, Patricia B. Sutker, *Comprehensive Handbook of Psychopathology* (2001).

109   **Our autonomic nervous system:** http://biologiedelapeau.fr/spip. php?article20.

109   **Nerve endings in our skin:** Lynn, B, Shahanbeh, J., "Substance P Content of The Skin, Neurogenic Inflammation And Numbers of C-Fibres Following Capsaicin Application To A Cutaneous Nerve In The Rabbit," *Neuroscience.* 1988 Mar;24(3):769-75.

**CHAPTER 6. SPEAKING THROUGH DREAMS**

121   **While role playing each different element:** Gestalt-annarbor.org/ Reading_Room/Perls%20Dream%20Interpretation.pdf.

121   **In many cases, this promotes:** Nevis, E. (2000) Introduction, in . *Gestalt Therapy: Perspectives and Applications.* Edwin Nevis (ed.). (Cambridge, MA: Gestalt Press), p. 3.

Latner, J. "The Theory of Gestalt Therapy," in *Gestalt Therapy: Perspectives and Applications*, Edwin Nevis (ed.) (Cambridge, MA: Gestalt Press, 2000).

Mackewn, J. *Developing Gestalt Counselling*. (London, UK: Sage Publications, 1997).

Bowman, C. & Brownell, P., "Prelude to Contemporary Gestalt Therapy," Gestalt!, vol. 4, no. 3, (2000), available at http://www.g-gej. org/4-3/prelude.html.

Leslie Grennberg and Philip Brownell, "Validating Gestalt. An Interview with Researcher, Writer, and Psychotherapist Leslie Greenberg," in Gestalt!, 1/1997.[1].

130   **A mechanical engineer named Mosche Feldenkrais:** http://www. feldenkrais.com/moshe-feldenkrais.

136   **His work suggests that the imagery:** http://www.nytimes. com/1984/07/10/science/do-dreams-really-contain-important-secret-meaning.html?pagewanted=all.

139   **When we observe ourselves performing a physical act:** Cannon, Walter (December 1927). "The James-Lange Theory of Emotions: A Critical Examination and an Alternative Theory," *The American Journal of Psychology* 39: 106–124. doi:10.2307/1415404.

Dalgleish, T., "The Emotional Brain" (PDF). *Nature Reviews Neuroscience* 5 (7) (2004). : 583–589. doi:10.1038/nrn1432. PMID 15208700.

George, M. S., Nahas, Z., Bohning, D. E., Kozel, F. A., Anderson, B.; et al. (2002). "Vagus Nerve Stimulation Therapy: A Research Update." Neurology 59 (6 supplement 4): S56–S61. doi:10.1212/wnl.59.6_suppl_4.s56.

Prinz, J. (2004), "Emotions Embodied," in Solomon, R., *Thinking about Feeling: Contemporary Philosophers on Emotions* (PDF). (Oxford University Press, 2011). pp. 44–59.

Redding, Paul, "Feeling, Thought, and Orientation: William James and the Idealist Anti-Cartesian Tradition," (PDF). *Parrhesia Journal* 13 (2011): 41–51.

Lang, Peter J. "The Varieties of Emotional Experience: A Meditation on James–Lange Theory." *Psychological Review* 101 (2) 1994: 211–221. doi:10.1037/0033-295x.101.2.211.

Ellsworth, P. C., "William James and Emotion: Is a Century of Fame Worth a Century of Misunderstanding?" *Psychological Review* 101 (2) 1994: 222–229. doi:10.1037/0033-295x.101.2.222Feldman.

Barrett, Lisa (2012). "Emotions are Real." American Psychological Association 12 (3): 413–429. doi:10.1037/a0027555.

Gross, James J., Lisa Feldman Barrett, "Emotion Generation and Emotion Regulation: One or Two Depends on Your Point of View." *Emotion Review* 3 (1) 2011: 816. doi:10.1177/1754073910380974.

Johnsen, E.L., Tranel, D., Lutgendorf, S., Adolphs, R. "A Neuroanatomical Dissociation for Emotion Induced by Music," *Emotion Review* 72 (1) 2009: 24–33. doi:10.1016/j.ijpsycho.2008.03.011. PMC 265 6600. PMID 18824047.

142   **Once depression sets in:** Robert Dantzer, Jason C. O'Connor, Gregory G. Freund, Rodney W. Johnson, and Keith W. Kelley, "From Inflammation to Sickness and Depression: When the Immune System Subjugates the Brain, *Nat Rev Neurosci.* 2008 Jan; 9(1): 46–56. http://www.apa.org/research/action/immune.aspx.

142   **Many people feel discomfort in an around the head. . . .** Means-Christensen, A., et al., "Relationships Among Pain, Anxiety, and Depression in Primary Care." *Depression and Anxiety 0:1-8* (2007).

de Filippis, S., Salvatori E., Coloprisco, G., Martelletti, P., "Headache and Mood Disorders," *J Headache Pain.* 2005 Sep;6(4):250-3.

http://www.health.harvard.edu/mind-and-mood/depression_and_pain.

Cui-Bai Wei, Jian-Ping Jia, Fen Wang, Ai-Hong Zhou, Xiu-Mei Zuo, and Chang-Biao Chu, "Overlap between Headache, Depression, and Anxiety" in "General Neurological Clinics: A Cross-sectional Study," *Chin Med J* (Engl). 2016 Jun 20; 129(12): 1394–1399.

## CHAPTER 7: CONVERSATIONS IN NATURE

146   **This belief is supported by many psychologists:** Theodore Millon, Melvin J. Lerner, Irving B. Weiner, *Handbook of Psychology, Personality, and Social Psychology,* 2003 .

156   **Despite the fact that about one in ten:** http://www.nimh.nih.gov/about/director/2011/antidepressants-a-complicated-picture.shtml.

http://www.ncbi.nlm.nih.gov/pmc/articles/PMC181155/table/i1523-5998-003-01-0022-t02/.

## CHAPTER 8: A DRAWING WORTH TEN THOUSAND WORDS

164   **Dr. Cathy Malchiodi, a pioneering child therapist:** Malchiodi, C.,
*Breaking the Silence: Art Therapy with Children from Violent Homes* (Bruner/
Mazel Publishers, 1997).

## CHAPTER 9: A DIALOGUE WITH DEATH

191   **It gives you an opportunity to feel good:** Clifton Bryant, *The Handbook of
Death and Dying,* (SAGE Publications, Inc; 1 edition, 2003).

196   **But recent medical research suggests:** http://www.cancer.gov/about-
cancer/coping/feelings/stress-fact-sheet.

Cohen, L et al., "Depressive Symptoms and Cortisol Rhythmicity Predict
Survival in Patients with Renal Cell Carcinoma: Role of Inflammatory
Signaling," 2012, http://dx.doi.org/10.1371/journal.pone.0042324.

http://thechart.blogs.cnn.com/2010/06/08/embargoed-68-less-stress-
helps-breast-cancer-patients/.

# INDEX

211

## ABOUT THE AUTHORS

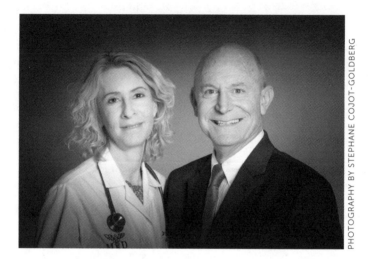

### DR. CHRIS GILBERT

Dr. Chris Gilbert is an Integrative and Holistic Medicine physician MD, PhD, now focusing mostly on public speaking. For fifteen years, she was in private practice in California, specializing in the combination of Western and Eastern Medicine and dedicating her life to treating and curing symptoms and illnesses that other physicians haven't been able to address. She is known for her exceptional success in treating chronic fatigue syndrome, anxiety, depression, recurrent infections, lower back pain, sexual problems, unexplained abdominal pain, and arthritis through methods she pioneered (described in detail in this book).

Before establishing her private practice, Dr. Gilbert worked with Doctors Without Borders and treated a staggering variety of illness suffered by poor and displaced people around the world. She has worked with patients in Mozambique (a pediatric hospital during a civil war), Sri Lanka (28,000 refugees in the north of the Island during a civil war), Mauritania (Touareg refugee camp at the border of Mali) and China (400,000 people displaced by floods). She is an active member of Doctors Without Borders.

Prior to those assignments, she was in a private medical practice in Paris, France, for seven years.

Dr. Gilbert holds a General Medicine MD and PhD from Cochin Medical School in Paris, France, and certifications in Hyperbaric Medicine, Sexology, Acupuncture, and Homeopathy. She is licensed in California, interned at University of California, Irvine, and served her residency at Harbor-UCLA Medical Center. She serves at times as a medical adviser for TV shows such as CSY NY.

In 2010 she self-published two books that she sold to her patients: *Dr. Chris's A, B, C's of Health* and *The French Stethoscope (a memoir)*.

She is a co-blogger with her husband Dr. Haseltine, on PsychologyToday.com

## DR. ERIC HASELTINE

Eric Haseltine is a neuroscientist with over thirty years experience applying advances in brain research to everyday problems. He has used his skills in fields as diverse as brain research, aerospace, entertainment, and national security.

He holds a PhD in Physiological Psychology from Indiana University and completed postdoctoral training in Neuroanatomy at Vanderbilt Medical School.

His current research focuses on mind-body interactions. He has written over one hundred articles on the brain for *Discover* magazine and Discovermagazine.com as well as sixty-five articles on applied neuroscience at PsychologyToday.com.

Haseltine drew on his training as a brain scientist to author or coauthor twenty-one issued patents and twenty-three pending patents.

In his 2010 book *Long Fuse Big Bang*, Dr. Haseltine showed how to apply principles of neuroscience to accelerating innovation.

He served as the head of Research and Development at both The Walt Disney Company and The National Security Agency. In his last government post from 2005-2007, he was the Director of Science and Technology for the entire U.S. Intelligence community.